The 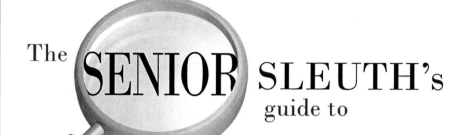 SENIOR SLEUTH's
guide to

Technology *for* Seniors

by David Peterka

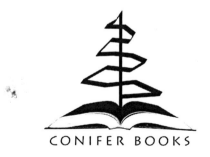

CONIFER BOOKS

Senior Sleuth's Guide to Technology for Seniors
Published by
Conifer Books, LLC
9599 South Turkey Creek Road
Morrison, CO 80465
www.coniferbooks.com
Copyright © 2009 by Conifer Books

Visit us at www.sleuthguides.com for more sleuthing topics.

ISBN: 978-0-9825652-0-9
Printed in the United States of America.

About the Author

David Peterka is a technology writer who provides technical (and other) support for his senior parents. David is the founder of the Senior Sleuth Guides and produces the online senior sleuthing website. Check out his latest work by visiting www.sleuthguides.com.

Author's Acknowledgements

I acknowledge that Claudia, Vern, Bob and Kitty are sweet parents and great sports for participating in all of my crazy senior schemes. I also acknowledge that Kristen has superhuman patience and extends a level of support that sometimes makes me question her judgment. She is the sweetest of all.

Thanks also to the many others who helped in some way with this book including Uncle Doctor Bob, Amy, Josh, Mandy, Ray, Nick, and the notorious Scott.

Dedication

To the curious senior who learns just because. I like you.

What one man can invent another can discover.

—Sherlock Holmes
The Adventure of the Dancing Man

Contents at a Glance

Table of Contents

The Case of Senior Technology

Senior Sleuth Case File #12995

Companies churn out thousands of new gadgets each year: from new automobile engines to button-sized music players that can store your entire music collection (and then some). Every time you blink ten strange new technologies pop up in casual conversation.

"I'm thinking about upgrading my laptop," your son says.

No problem. You're hanging in there. But then he continues...

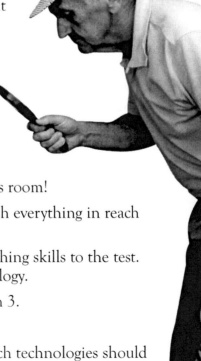

"I'm looking at a 2.53 gigahertz Intel Core Duo P8700 processor running on Vista with 4 gigabyte dual channel SDRAM at 1067 megahertz. Of course I'll want wireless N."

Your head is now spinning at a dangerous rate. You consider your three options:

1. Plug your ears, start humming your favorite Sinatra tune, and order your adult son to go to his room!

2. Grab a hammer and smash everything in reach with a blinking light.

3. Investigate. Put your sleuthing skills to the test. Learn more about technology.

You, of course, choose option 3.

You are on the case!

But where do you start? Which technologies should you research? After ten seconds of deliberation, the answer is obvious. You start by learning about the technology that will best serve you—Technology for Seniors.

After another ten seconds, you realize that this is still a fairly big bite to swallow—Senior Technology is an enormous topic! Senior Technology is not limited to gadgets with "for Seniors" on the label. This broad technology category includes anything that can make senior life more graceful, independent, invigorating, and fun.

For example, most of us don't think of high-speed Internet as a Senior Technology. Most of us, at least in this case, are wrong. The Internet is the quintessential Senior Technology! It allows seniors to manage and share health records with doctors and caregivers, research and book the next international trip, foster relationships with kids and grandkids through social networking sites, and continue self-education by researching any conceivable topic from the comfort of their own home. The Internet enriches the senior experience; it is therefore a Senior Technology!

So it's decided. You will investigate the most pervasive Senior Technologies— from the Internet to gadgets for longer independent living.

Your first stop in the investigation is— you guessed it—this book. You grab your reading glasses, pour yourself a glass of brandy, and turn the page.

You are on the case! Learn about technologies that will enrich the Senior experience.

The Profile: What is a Senior Sleuth?

You are!

You were curious about something. You bought a book. And now you're sleuthing.

A Senior Sleuth is any senior citizen curious enough about a particular topic to investigate. Although learning any new topic or skill can be daunting at first, the Senior Sleuth knows that patience and persistence will crack the toughest case.

In fact, as a Senior Sleuth you have an advantage over younger investigators. You have a full lifetime of experiences. This will help you more easily contextualize new concepts—comparing them to another of your billion life experiences—so that the new fits nicely in with the old.

For example: You hear of this gadget called a Global Positioning System (GPS) device, which maps your exact location, no matter where you are. This immediately makes sense to you. You, like every other person on the planet, sometimes get lost while driving or hiking an unfamiliar trail. In fact, you've gone more places (and have subsequently gotten more lost) than younger folks, so you understand the need for this device better than most. You might not know how it works or how to use the thing, but you now know the technology exists and you have the option to learn more.

But, of course, you already know this. That's why you are here. I'll stop yammering. It's time to investigate.

Investigative Tools: About this Book

This book provides an overview, detailed at times, of today's most pervasive and helpful Senior Technologies. It is organized into the following sections:

✓ Computers

✓ Internet

✓ Health and medication management

✓ Tools for longer independent living

✓ Communication devices for keeping in touch

✓ Travel and transportation

✓ Home Entertainment

✓ Futuristic stuff

I'm not going to go into detail about how to use this book. You are a Senior Sleuth for goodness' sake! You already know how to use a table of contents and index, so spending time here would just delay your investigation.

I will, however, offer one investigative clue. Each section of this book is self-contained, so if you are only curious about, say, online shopping, then skip to Chapter 3. There is no need to read from front cover to back. And even if there were a need, I couldn't make you do it. The Senior Sleuth is a stubborn creature who will do as he or she pleases. As well you should!

Oh, just one more thing...

Throughout this book you'll see the following graphic icons highlighting things I think are important or interesting.

Clue	Hints for learning more about a particular topic. These can be Web search terms or supporting information that you could find helpful.
Tip-off	Tips on performing some action or learning more about a particular topic.
Modus operandi	Instructions for performing some task. This could be steps for navigating a complex television remote or advice on purchasing a new TV from an online vendor.
Just the facts	Strange and wonderful facts about a particular piece of technology. These could be quirky historical tidbits or even quirkier present-day uses of the technology.
Who dunnit?	Famous characters or companies associated with a given technology.
Watch it!	Warning. Danger. Don't be a hero. Forget the Alamo. Be careful!

The Rise of Senior Technology

N eed and want. These are the driving forces of innovation, the carrot and stick that motivate industry to develop new gadgets and gizmos. The more people that need or want technologies, the quicker those technologies come to market.

Enter the Baby Boomer generation.

According to the U.S. Census Bureau, the Baby Boomer generation includes 78 million people born in the US between 1946 and 1964. In 2006, the oldest of this generation turned sixty years old. On average, 7000 US citizens will turn sixty each day through 2026.

What does this mean?

It means that the number of consumers of Senior Technology is growing at a fantastic rate. Consequently, industry is racing to gain market share and develop technologies for that demographic.

Not only is there a huge number of boomers entering the Senior Technology market, senior consumers are uniquely attractive to industry. Why? Seniors have money and they spend it.

As the growing senior community needs and wants more technology for their unique situations and lifestyles, industry will race to feed it to them.

In this chapter you will investigate:

➤ Senior Technology Market

➤ Things You Didn't Have When You Were a Kid

➤ Aging-In-Place Technologies

➤ Senior Technology Categories

Senior Technology Market

The Senior Technology market is exploding.

Thousands of companies are getting into the Senior Technology market each year. Industry giants like IBM, Microsoft, and Google are actively enhancing their healthcare and elder offerings to attract aging consumers. Professional coalitions dedicated to the development of Senior Technologies are expanding their memberships.

For example, The Center for Aging Services Technologies (CAST) now consists of over 400 technology companies, service organizations and research institutions, each working to "expedite the development, evaluation and adoption of emerging technologies that will transform the aging experience." [CAST Website]

Industry has finally noticed the senior market.

In 2009, the International Consumer Electronics Show (CES)—the largest such trade show in the world—featured a number of Senior Technologies in their Silvers Summit.

As the demand for Senior Technologies grows, expect to see more companies offering more products to the senior community.

JUST THE FACTS

Senior Wealth

+ 78 million Americans who were 50 or older as of 2001 controlled 67% of the country's wealth, or $28 trillion (U.S. Census and Federal Reserve).

+ Households headed by someone between the ages 55 and 64 had a median net worth of $112,048 in 2000—15 times greater than the under 35 age group (U.S. Census and Federal Reserve).

+ Americans 50 and older have $2.4 trillion in annual income, which accounts for 42% of all after-tax income (U.S. Consumer Expenditure Survey).

Senior Spending

+ Americans 50 and older account for an estimated $2 trillion in total expenditures for 2005.

+ $2.3 trillion in disposable income.

+ Between now and 2010, the total spending for 50+ households will increase by over $900 billion.

+ In 2004, people aged 50 and older spent an average of 47.6 percent of their family's budget on "nonessentials" (Bureau of Labor).

When I was a Kid, We Didn't Have…

As you begin your investigation into Senior Technology, one fact quickly smacks you in the face—all of the recent world-changing technologies were conceived of and developed during your lifetime! You witnessed the birth of high-tech.

I know this sounds like the premise to a classic joke, but your list of "I didn't have that when I was a kid," is truly amazing. Let's take a look at some of the biggies that appeared in just the last few decades.

Home Computers

Home computers were developed in the late 1970's, gained widespread popularity in the 1980's, and have since found their way into over 75% of American homes. We use these for everything: word processing, playing games, communication (email and the Internet), shopping, business management, and education—to name a few.

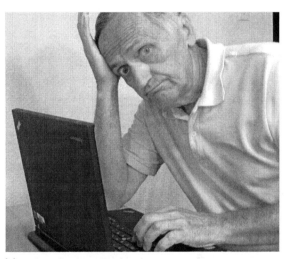

More seniors are using computers.

Digital Cameras

Photography is now accessible to the casual user. We can snap a picture, immediately see it on a digital display, and then upload it to our computer. From there we can touch it up and print it—all without access to a darkroom full of chemicals. Of course, you still need to have an eye for photography to get a good picture.

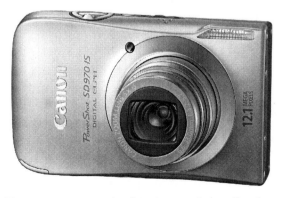

Tiny cameras can display pictures immediately.

Internet

This global network of computers has revolutionized how we exchange information. We can now send emails, photographs, and other large collections of digital information from the comfort of our home computer. The amount of information at our fingertips is mind-blowing.

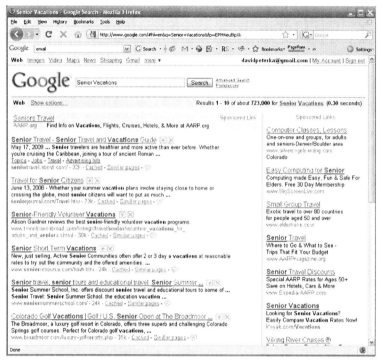

Volumes of information and entertainment at your fingertips.

Portable Music Players

Now you can listen to your favorite music while strolling down the street. Simply clip the player to your shirt, place the nearly invisible speakers in your ears, and enjoy!

Tiny devices like the one shown here can hold ALL of your music library.

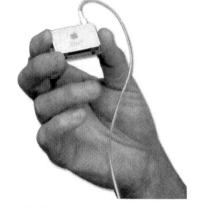

iPod shuffle music player.

Cell Phones

We thought in-home cordless phones were neat. Well, they were—but cell phones are even neater. Now you can stay in touch with friends and family from just about anywhere in the world (at least anywhere relatively close to a cell tower). The latest generation of cell phones has gotten even neater. Phones, like the Apple iPhone, include Internet access, music players, cameras, and mapping technologies.

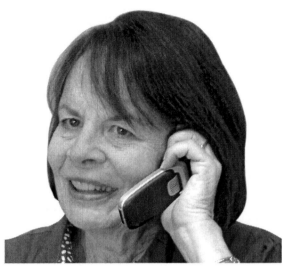

Cell phones keep us in touch no matter where we go.

Robot Vacuum Cleaners

Although I include this item in jest, they really do exist, and it does illuminate a world of possibilities. Don't like vacuuming—who does?—get a robot to do it. It won't be long before we have robots to wash our dishes, shovel our driveways, and paint our houses. Is this going to make us lazy? Maybe, but it will be fascinating to find out!

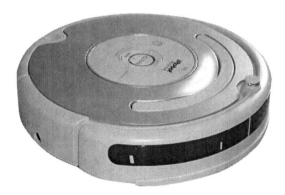

The Roomba robot will clean your floor and then recharge itself.

This is just a small sample of the new consumer technology available to all of us. We will go into more detail on these and other technological advancements in later chapters.

Aging In Place Technologies

We want to be comfortable. We want to be surrounded by familiar things and people. We want to grow old in our own homes. We want to age in place.

Age-In-Place technology refers specifically to the gadgets that help you live independently in your own home longer. This includes health and medication management, home monitoring devices, and communication tools to stay connected with friends and family.

More and more seniors are aging in place with the help of advanced technologies and better home ergonomics. For example, you can now buy sensors for your home that will detect falls or long periods of inactivity and then notify family (via phone or Internet) when something seems wrong.

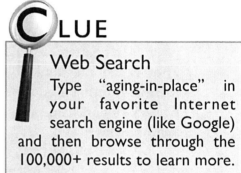

CLUE

Web Search
Type "aging-in-place" in your favorite Internet search engine (like Google) and then browse through the 100,000+ results to learn more.

Other Senior Technology Categories

Senior Technology refers to a broad range of gadgets and gizmos that help improve the lives of seniors—from aging-in-place tools to new forms of entertainment to websites for finding and booking great travel deals.

Remember that a product does not need to have the label "for Seniors" to be a Senior Technology.

Here are the Senior Technologies that we'll investigate in this book:

✓ Computers

✓ Internet

✓ Health and medication management

✓ Tools for longer independent living

✓ Communication devices for keeping in touch

✓ Travel and transportation

✓ Home Entertainment

✓ Futuristic stuff

Should We Categorize Senior Technology?

Wait just one minute! If we're calling any technology that enhances senior life "Senior Technology," then is there really a distinction between Modern Technology and Senior Technology? Also, is the industry condescending to seniors by marketing directly to them?

Good questions, Senior Sleuth! Let's investigate the differing viewpoints.

Argument AGAINST Senior Technology Classification

We should NOT label things Senior Technologies. By classifying something as a Senior Technology, you set the senior community apart from the rest of consumers. Sure, we seniors are a little older than you, but we have similar interests and needs as younger generations. We want to be treated like everyone else. Calling something a Senior Technology places a negative connotation on the product and seniors, suggesting that seniors need more help and more technology than everyone else.

Argument FOR Senior Technology Classification

We should absolutely have our own category of products and technologies. We are a large and powerful demographic with unique needs and interests, and we're willing to pay for items that are designed for us. I'm proud to be called a Senior. I've spent a lot of time earning the title, and now that I have it I want it to mean something positive. Slap the "Senior Technology" label on anything that will help me live better so it's easier for me to identify, buy and enjoy.

So, which argument is correct?

I invite you to form your own opinion. In the meantime, here is mine.

The Senior Technology label should be applied to anything that meets the following requirements: 1) it helps enhance the senior's life, and 2) it does so through features, which target the unique needs of the older generation (considering such needs as social, economic, health and ergonomic).

So, a car wouldn't be classified as a Senior Technology because it only meets the first requirement—it enhances their lives—but fails the second requirement because it does not (on the whole) offer features specifically addressing senior usability concerns. However, a voice GPS navigation device inside the car would meet both requirements—it enhances life by offering directions AND has senior-friendly voice features that allow the senior traveler to more easily get to his or her destination.

It's a fuzzy area, I know. You could argue almost any technology into the Senior Technology category. For example, a wide-handled toothbrush could easily squeeze into this category—it improves dental health and is easier for arthritic hands to grasp.

For the purposes of this investigation, we'll limit Senior Technologies to modern or cutting-edge tools that address senior challenges related to health, independent living, communication, and entertainment.

Home Computers

O ne of the first stops in your Senior Technology investigation will be your bedroom or den. This is where you probably keep your home computer.

Don't have a computer?

Then you are in the minority. According to a 2003 survey by the US Census Bureau, 62% of the households in the US have a computer in their home. Over 54% of homes had Internet access. And this was in 2003! Since then computer prices have fallen and Internet access is faster and cheaper than ever.

True, seniors are a little behind the home computing curve, with only about 40% of senior households with a home computer, according to a 2006 Census Bureau survey. But this is quickly changing. More seniors are getting home computers or laptops each day.

There's a good reason that so many Americans have a computer in their home. Computers allow everyone (not just Senior Sleuths) to access the Internet and countless software applications that enrich our lives.

But which computers are more senior friendly—PCs or Macs? Who can fix your computer when there is a problem? Which software programs do you need?

Great questions, Senior Sleuth. Let's go find some answers.

In this chapter you will investigate:

➢ Computer Terminology

➢ Operating System Considerations for Seniors

➢ Which is better for you: Laptop or Desktop?

➢ Should you buy a "Senior PC?"

➢ Senior Software

➢ Remote Help for Computer Problems

➢ Computer Security

Background Check

With new ways to shop, interactive games, faster communication, and new business opportunities, the home computer (coupled with the Internet) has changed the very fabric of American life. And the most amazing thing is the timing—this all happened during our watch, in just the last few decades.

Check out this high-level timeline to see some major milestones in home computing.

(Sorry for the tiny font. This would be a great time to pull out your Senior Sleuthing spyglass.)

1950

1954
Commodore founded as a typewriter company.

1955
Steve Jobs (Apple founder) and Bill Gates (Microsoft founder) born.

1969
UNIX Operating System is developed at AT&T's Bell Labs.

1972
Atari ships Pong, the first video game.
C computer language developed at Bell Labs.

1975
Bill Gates and Paul Allen found Microsoft.

1976
Steve Jobs and Steve Wozniak build first Apple computer (Apple I).

1977
Radio Shack releases TRS-80 computer with keyboard, video display, and tape cassette.

1981
IBM PC released with Microsoft's DOS operating system.
250,000 computers sold!

1982
Over 3 million computers sold!

1984
Apple releases the Macintosh computer, featuring a graphical interface.

1988
Microsoft becomes the largest software vendor.

1989
Intel creates a chip with more than one million transistors.

1995
Microsoft releases Windows 95.
Sun launches Java, popular programming language for Internet apps.

1996
Two out of three employees in the US use a PC.

1997
Intel creates chip with 7.5 million transistors.
DVDs created.
Deep Blue beats Kasparov in chess.

1998
eCommerce (internet businesses) booms.

2001
Windows XP released.
Apple launches iPod.

2002
One billionth computer sold!

2007
Two billionth computer sold!

2010

Computer Terminology

Computers are getting more user friendly each year, but there are still a few confusing concepts and terms. Don't worry, though—once you get the hang of the basic terminology, computers are manageable. This section defines the common components of a modern computer system.

Computer Tower

This is the main body of the computer where all of the processing happens. Here are the main components that comprise the computer tower:

✓ **Hard drive**—Device that stores data even when not powered. This allows us to turn off the computer and maintain our data and computer settings.

✓ **Memory (also called RAM)**—Form of data storage, which allows the data to be accessed in any order (or at random). This memory is erased when the computer is shut off. More RAM means that your computer will process data more quickly.

✓ **Processor (Central Processing Unit, or CPU)**—This is the brain of the computer. It's "speed" is measured in frequency range (hertz). The higher the number, the faster and more powerful the computer.

✓ **Operating System (OS)**—The interface between the hardware and the software. The two most popular consumer operating systems are Windows and Mac OS.

✓ **Software**—Computer programs that perform tasks on a computer. These range from word processors to computer games.

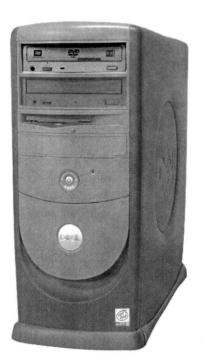

The computer tower holds the "guts" of the computer.

✓ **Ports**—The outlets on the computer, which are used to connect external devices such as the keyboard, mouse, or printer. These are typically found on the rear of the computer, although some ports (like the USB for attaching devices such as digital cameras) are often located on the front.

Monitor

Visual display device where you can see what is happening in the computer. Make sure to read reviews of different monitors before purchasing one. There are wide variations in quality and sizes.

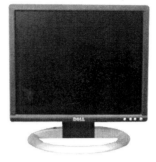

Monitor

Keyboard

Input device modeled after the typewriter. Alternate "ergonomic" keyboards are available to help avoid repetitive stress injuries.

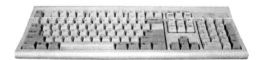

Keyboard

Mouse

Device for pointing at and selecting objects on your computer screen. A variety of mouse designs are available to help avoid repetitive stress caused by prolific use of the device.

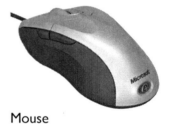

Mouse

Modem (with Wireless)

Device for sending and receiving data over the Internet. Modems typically get their signals from a phone or cable line and then translate that signal into something the computer can understand. Modems can be connected to your computer via a cable or wireless signals.

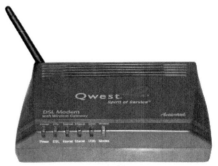

Modem for connecting to the Internet

Printer (laser or inkjet)

Device for printing text or pictures from your computer. Use laser printers when you want to print a lot of text quickly. Use inkjets for higher quality photo prints.

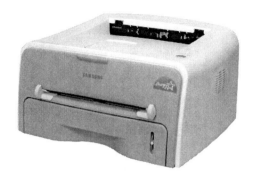

Laser Printer

Webcam

Device for capturing and sending video from your computer. These are typically placed on top of the computer monitor or on your desk. This is a must-have device if you want to have a "video chat" with a friend.

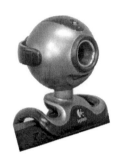

Webcam

Put all of these pieces together and you are ready for some major computing!

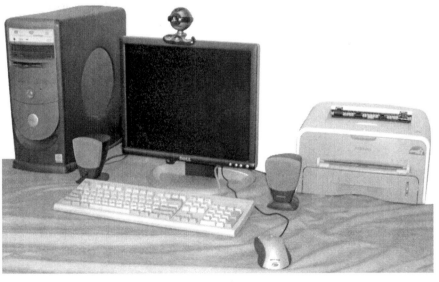

Home Computer System Setup

Operating Systems (Microsoft Windows Versus Mac)

If you wander into a debate over which is the best operating system, you'll probably witness two enthusiastic maniacs exchanging blows on their system's reliability (which system crashes less frequently) and usability (which system is easier to learn and navigate). Tread lightly if you enter into one of these debates. Some people are passionate about their operating systems.

The two main consumer operating systems are Microsoft Windows and Mac OS. The Windows operating system runs on a "PC," which is a generic term for any computer running on the Microsoft Windows operating system. PC computers are manufactured from dozens of different companies such as Dell and IBM. The Mac OS is only run on Mac computers.

Reliability and Service

Mac devotees argue that the Mac is more reliable (i.e. less prone to "crashing," or unexpected shut-downs) than PCs. But is the Mac always more reliable? Does Apple have the best customer service on the market? Well... yes and no. According to a 2008 Consumer Reports survey of laptop computers, two machines consistently came out on top: the Mac (from Apple) and Lenovo (which can run Windows). Lenovo actually scored better than the Macs for reliability. On the flip side, the Mac scored better than Lenovo for customer service.

The Lenovo, of course, is only one out of a dozen manufactures using the Windows operating system. So though you can not claim that the Mac is always better than the PC, a solid argument can be made that the Mac is usually more reliable than the PC.

WHO DUNNIT?

Bill Gates is the infamous founder of Microsoft—the company responsible for the Microsoft Windows operating system. Bill Gates was worth $58 billion in 2008.

Steve Jobs is the co-founder and latest CEO of Apple—the company responsible for the Mac operating system (as well as the iPod and iPhone products). Steve Jobs was worth roughly $6 billion in 2008.

Mac Pros and Cons

Mac PROs:

✛ The PC World website has given the Mac top scores for service and reliability. If you buy a Mac, then you can be relatively sure that you have purchased a quality machine. And if you by unlikely chance buy a lemon, Apple's customer service will take care of you.

✛ The Mac operating system and machine both come from the same company, so you are less likely to experience strange compatibility software issues. If you buy software for your Mac, it will work on your Mac.

✛ Macs are less likely to be targeted by software viruses. Windows has historically been the target of most computer attacks because they hold the majority of the market—not because they are poorly designed.

Mac CONs:

■ Less flexibility with features and prices compared to Windows. You will probably pay more for a Mac.

■ Some software only runs on Windows.

■ Less people use it. This last point is actually a pretty big negative for the senior user—especially if you expect occasional help from friends, neighbors, or children. If they don't use a Mac, then they won't be able to help you with any of your technical (or non-technical) problems.

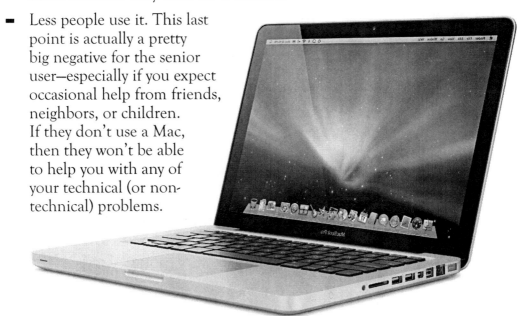

Mac laptop computer. (Photo courtesy of Apple)

Windows Pros and Cons:

Windows PROs:

✛ Some PCs and Laptops running Windows score very high in the reliability and service department.

✛ Thousands of computer configurations available from hundreds of PC distributors and manufacturers. This allows you to pick a machine that is right for your processing level and pocketbook.

✛ Supports virtually all software applications. (More companies develop software for the Windows platform.)

✛ More people use Windows, and so getting support from friends and family will be easier.

Windows CONs:

– Some PCs and Laptops running Windows score very LOW in the reliability and service department. When purchasing a PC, you need to research the different companies and their products. Consumer Reports is one good way to research products before buying them. You can also check www.cnet.com for reviews.

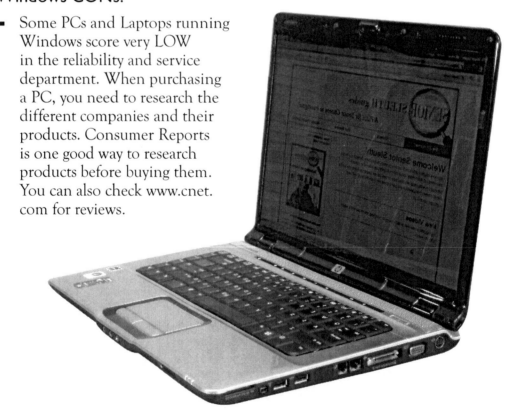

Windows laptop computer.

Senior-Friendly Features (Mac vs. Windows)

The latest incarnations of the Mac and Windows operating systems both include "accessibility" features, which help users with special needs. For example, the Mac operating system includes VoiceOver, which reads the screen to those users with limited eyesight. Windows includes a similar feature (Narrator) through its accessibility screen.

Additionally, both operating systems allow you to change the display font sizes for easier reading, and support integration with other senior-friendly peripherals, such as larger navigation touch pads.

As of this printing, neither operating system is considerably more accessible than the other.

So, Which Operating System Wins for Seniors?

Neither the Windows nor Mac operating system is the clear winner on the Senior Technology front. Both support accessibility features and applications, and both can (depending on the PC manufacturer) score well in reliability and service.

Make sure to research company and product before buying any PC. Unlike Macs, which are famously reliable, some PC manufacturers create shoddy products and have even worse service.

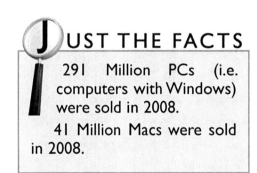

JUST THE FACTS

291 Million PCs (i.e. computers with Windows) were sold in 2008.

41 Million Macs were sold in 2008.

You don't have to fall into the trap of "I already know Windows, so I can't learn Mac." This simply isn't true. It will take a few days to get the hang of a new operating system, but then you'll be just as proficient as you were with Windows—maybe more so.

Remember to consider your support lines. If you plan to turn to your friends and family for computer help, you need to get the same operating system that they have. This, more often than not, means you should buy a PC.

Modus Operandi

How to turn on Microsoft Windows Narrator

Windows Narrator reads the Windows elements from your computer screen.

To turn on Microsoft Windows Narrator:

1. Turn on your computer.

2. Click the **Start** button in the lower left hand corner of the computer screen.

3. Use your mouse to move the pointer over the following menu items in this sequence: **All Programs > Accessories > Accessibility > Narrator.**

4. Click on **Narrator**.

Microsoft Narrator will then begin speaking to you. Make sure you have your computer speakers turned on in order to hear the voice. Note that Narrator reads the names of windows, fields, and buttons, but does NOT read text in documents or web pages. If you need that level of narration, you will need to purchase a premium software.

See the "Text to Speech" software section on page 31 for more information.

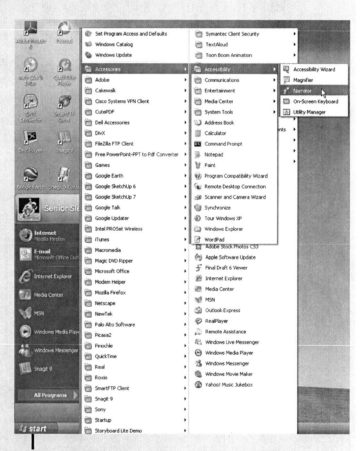

Click **Start > All Programs > Accessories > Accessibility > Narrator.**

Laptops Versus Desktops

The latest generation of laptops offers processing speeds and reliability on par with their desktop counterparts. Let's quickly compare laptops and desktops to see if one is better for the senior community on the whole.

Price	Laptops cost more. To get a laptop with equivalent processing power as a desktop, you could pay twice as much (or more). But don't let this discourage you from the laptop altogether. Both desktop and laptop prices are falling, so neither purchase is going to break the bank. Also, who says you need equivalent processing power—why not get a slightly slower laptop and save yourself some cash?
	As of this printing, you could get a barebones desktop (including monitor, keyboard, and mouse) for $500. I also saw a few laptops (from a good company) for under $600.
Storage	Desktops usually come with larger hard drives, which can store more information. If you use your computer for intense photo applications or video editing, then you need a lot of storage space.
	Laptops can have a lot of storage, but they cost more.
Graphics and Games	Are you a hardcore video gamer? If so, the desktop wins again. Desktops typically come with better graphic cards and can be easily upgraded if you ever need better graphics.
	Again, laptops can come with better graphic capabilities, but this is expensive.
Screen Size	Desktops require a separate external monitor. You can therefore buy the monitor that fits your visual requirements. If you have poor eyesight, you'll want a bigger monitor.
	The largest laptop monitor is around 20 inches on the diagonal—which is pretty big for a portable device. Desktop monitors now come as large as 30 inches, which is bigger than any of our TVs were when we were kids.

Upgrading	Say you want more power, more storage space, a better video card. If you have a desktop, no problem—you can buy and install the hardware to support your decadent desires. If, however, you have a laptop, you can pretty much forget about it. Laptops are really difficult—if not impossible—to upgrade. For this reason, you probably should buy a more powerful laptop upfront so that it doesn't become obsolete within a year.
Portability	Finally, the laptop wins! This is why you get a laptop—so you can take it with you on your trip across the country, to the coffee shop, to your kid's house for free tech support.

In summary, desktops are cheaper, more powerful, and can be equipped with a larger monitor. However, you can take a laptop with you. If you want to use your computer away from your house, you need a laptop. If you don't travel or wouldn't take the computer with you if you did travel, then the desktop is a good bet.

CLUE

Web Search
Type "laptop versus desktop" into your favorite Web search engine and browse the thousands of search results.

The SeniorPC

Microsoft has recognized the senior market and has created the "Senior PC"—a computer specifically tailored to the senior community. These computers are preloaded with senior-friendly software (like medical and financial management applications) and include other senior-friendly options like larger keys on the keyboard (for the desktop) or easy-to-open latches (on the laptop). Some even include a meta-presentation-layer on top of the regular Windows operating system that further simplifies the most common computing tasks.

You can purchase the Senior PC (SeniorPC) through Microsoft's website at the following address: www.microsoft.com/enable/aging/seniorpc.aspx. They currently offer two models:

✓ **Standard:** Regular PC or laptop with preloaded helpful software. List price approximately $1200 (with options for additional senior-friendly accessories).

✓ **Autopilot:** This is the standard package plus additional features and software geared toward the senior user who is totally unfamiliar with computers. Most notably, this model features email, Internet, and word processing products by Qualilife—a company specializing in easy-to-use software for people with special needs. List price approximately $1300 (with options for additional senior-friendly accessories).

So now that you know these things exist, should you get one?

Maybe.

If you have never used a computer and break out into a cold sweat whenever you hear the word email, then you should consider it. The simplified email and Internet programs might be less intimidating, and could encourage you to explore other more advanced computer features. On the other hand, you are curious and savvy enough to read a book on technology, so who's to say you couldn't quickly learn how to use a regular computer?

If you currently have a computer or have successfully used one in the last few years, then you probably shouldn't bother. These SeniorPC configurations are more expensive than regular computers, and all they really do for you is install software they think you should have. You, Senior Sleuth, are perfectly capable of researching and loading whatever software you decide is right for a specific senior user—namely, you. You can still buy the oversized keyboard if you want, but I don't see a good reason for paying extra money for someone else to load software onto your machine.

Software for EVERYTHING

There is a computer program (or software) for everything: filing taxes, processing photographs, gaming, producing newsletters, creating websites, learning a language, and learning an instrument—to name only a few. If you have some sort of organizational, entertainment, or computational need, then there are probably already a dozen (or more) software programs that meet that need.

Don't believe me? Try this.

Think of something that you have needed to compute in the last six months and then type it into your favorite search engine. You'll be amazed with how many software programs are available—often for free!

Here's an example from my life. I was working on a small solar project at my house and needed to know how much solar radiation I could collect with a solar panel tilted at 30 degrees (the slope of my roof) facing South-south-east. A pretty obscure need, wouldn't you agree? I searched for the following terms in Google: `radiation solar collector angle`. The first search result was for a FREE program that would calculate what I needed based on my latitude and longitude. Perfect!

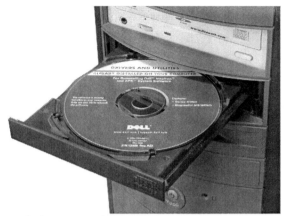

Software can be loaded onto your computer via CD or DVD disc.

We obviously can't investigate EVERY software out there. We can't even investigate every software out there targeted at seniors. So, we'll need to compromise. The following sections identify some consumer software in categories of interest to seniors AND will provide a few tips for selecting the best software for your needs.

Financial and Tax Software

Many seniors are on a fixed budget—the curse of blessed retirement. Tracking how much money you have today and will have tomorrow is an important strategy for living comfortably. Here are a few well-rated financial management software applications.

Each application is easy to install on any PC. They can be delivered either on CDs or you can download and install the programs from the vendor's website.

Financial Software: Intuit Quicken versus Microsoft Money

Financial management programs provide easy ways to consolidate, view and manage

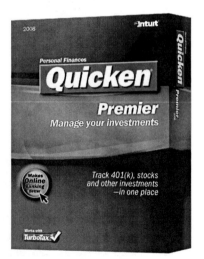

Quicken—a popular financial management software

your money. Select the Premier (for Quicken) or Premium (for Microsoft Money) editions of this software for more features for managing retirement investments.

Features	Both of these applications allow you to see all of your accounts in one place, track your retirement portfolio, analyze your spending, export data to your tax preparation software, and manage and pay your bills. Both also feature secure online transactions with your banks.
Cost on Amazon	Quicken Premier: $65.00 + shipping Microsoft Money Premium: $50.00 + shipping
Additional Costs:	You may need to upgrade periodically in order to maintain the link with your financial institutions. Upgrades typically cost less than the new license.

Recommendation: Both of these products are quite good, so there isn't a clear winner. Some surveys suggest that Quicken has a nicer interface and user experience. Also, Quicken utilizes a single secret PIN to access your financial data, whereas Microsoft Money requires you to use their Windows Live ID, which can be used by other applications, making it at least *feel* less secure. You'll need to decide if the bump in usability and added perception of security is worth an extra $15 to $20.

Tax Software: TurboTax and TaxCut

TurboTax (from Intuit, the same company that produces Quicken financial software) and TaxCut are both well-reviewed do-it-yourself tax programs. These programs prompt you to enter information from your W2s and other financial income, translate that information onto the official tax forms, calculate how much you owe or will get back, and check for errors.

Both of these applications also integrate with financial software (such as Quicken or Microsoft Money), allowing you to

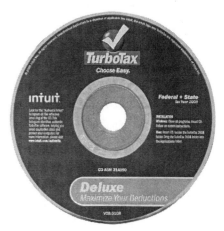

Turbotax—a popular tax preparation software

quickly import financial information from your computer.

The advantage to TaxCut is price. You can currently get the latest TaxCut on Amazon for around $30. TurboTax runs about $54.

The advantage to TurboTax is automatic downloads of W2s and other information from your financial institutions. TurboTax prompts you for the names of your employer and financial institutions and then downloads all of the information needed to fill out the income portions of your tax form. This saves time and reduces errors resulting from data entry mistakes.

Recommendation: If you're pressed for time and hate typing, choose TurboTax. If, however, you want to save $20 and love data entry, try TaxCut.

"Fun" Software to Sharpen Your Brain

Software gaming for seniors is a growing field. But senior games come with an added benefit—they make you smarter! Or they can at least slow cognitive decline.

It's a fact of life. Our brains get slower over time. And slower brains can lead to a host of other health (especially mental health) issues. So, to discourage cognitive decline, a few companies have devised computer games that help you stay mentally sharp.

Here are a few computer game recommendations (from `seniorjournal.com`).

Posit Science Brain Fitness Program

OK. Maybe this software isn't the most fun, and maybe it's not technically a game, but it will sharpen your brain. This software package was developed with the help of dozens of brain scientists. Their website boasts the following statistics:

✓ Ten year improvement in memory (meaning you will perform like someone ten years younger)

✓ 130% faster auditory processing speed

✓ 75% of users report that it has improved their lives

✓ Early studies show that this program

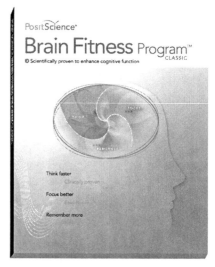

Brain Fitness package

can help those with early stages of Alzheimer's

This software includes six auditory exercises, each improving a different auditory or memory skill. By the end of the program, you will (according to Posit's website) be processing and memorizing certain auditory signals at a rate comparable to a 40-year-old. Not bad!

This is probably the most scientifically validated program out there. Unfortunately, all those clinical tests cost money, and so the price of the software is borderline outrageous. Amazon.com currently lists this program at just under $400. If you want a sharper brain, you might have to pay for the brain sharpener.

Posit Science Insight

Posit has developed a second software product that aims at improving the visual system: visual processing, visual precision (identifying and remembering visual queues), dividing visual attention (tracking other moving objects like other cars when driving), and visual memory.

Their website boasts the following statistics:

✓ 300% faster visual processing

✓ 200% better field of view

✓ Improved driving safety

Again, Posit really pushes the science behind their product. They need to do this to justify the cost, which is currently $400 on Amazon.com.

MindFit from CogniFit

MindFit is another software program scientifically validated to improve cognitive skills. Whereas the Posit Brain Fitness program focuses primarily on auditory skills, reaction time and memory, the MindFit program addresses a wide range of visual, auditory, response time and memory skills. As you improve, the exercises get more difficult, sharpening your brain with each session.

This program is still expensive, but it comes in at less than half the price of just one of the Posit programs. Amazon.com currently has MindFit listed at $140.

Dakim BrainFitness

Dakim offers a brain sharpening software and hardware combination. Their brain games are similar to other cognitive training systems, but they are only delivered with their own hardware. The hardware is really neat—featuring a touch screen for easy interaction. However, the hardware is also really expensive. For this reason, you'll only see these systems in homes of people with a lot of money or as a shared resource in a retirement or nursing facility.

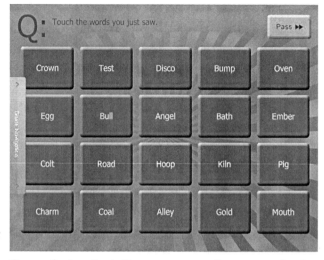

One of the BrainFitness games for strengthening memory. You must identify words that we shown on a previous screen. The game gets harder as you perform better.

The Dakim website doesn't actually list the price for their home system, but other resources on the Internet place the price at around $2,000. Yikes!

MyBrainTrainer.com

This online software program (meaning that you access it through a browser connected to the Internet) features a large number of fitness exercises. This program has not been subjected to as much scientific rigor as the other programs listed above, and it leans heavily on the "use it or lose it" philosophy of cognitive health. The site features tests, puzzles and games similar to the other brain fitness programs, so it's reasonable to expect similar brain sharpening results.

This software is accessible through a subscription, which equates to about $3 per month. If you don't mind forgoing the official scientific stamp of approval, you could check this out for a few months to see if it holds your interest and sharpens your brain. The cost is minimal and the potential benefit is great.

Special Needs and Accessibility Software

Accessibility software is a broad category of computer products for making your interaction with the computer easier. Currently the most prominent categories of accessibility software are:

✓ Text to Speech: Software that reads text on your screen, thus helping users with limited or no sight.

✓ Magnifiers: Software that allows you to magnify different parts of your screen, thus helping users with poor or failing eyesight.

✓ Speech Recognition: Software that allows you to interact with the computer using your voice, thus reducing keyboard and mouse dependence. This helps users with fine motor issues (e.g., users with Parkinson's Disease or Arthritis).

✓ Task simplification: Software that uses a simpler screen to perform basic computing tasks, such as sending emails or surfing the Internet.

Although the latest Windows and Mac operating systems are delivered with these types of accessibility programs (with the exception of task simplification... unless you opt to purchase the Microsoft SeniorPC), you can still purchase additional accessibility software from a third party.

But should you spend money when you can get similar features for free?

Maybe. Simply put, these for-purchase software packages are more robust than the features delivered with the operating system. If you depend on any of these features for a positive computer experience, then you should buy the software.

Below are a few different software programs in each of the above software accessibility categories.

Text to Speech

These software programs read items on your computer screen—from the names of windows to the body of an email or other document. But you need to manage your expectations here a bit. The voice will not be a deep booming James Earl Jones or a strong, character-rich Katharine Hepburn. Far from it. The voice will be an almost normal sounding voice, with a tinge of robot accent. Add to the strange synthetic nature of the voice its imperfect dramatic inflection or timing, and you have a recipe for a rather dull read.

Text-to-speech programs are not about pleasure reading—they are about accessibility. If having someone (or something) read aloud what's on the computer screen allows you to use the computer, then it has done its job. The following programs will read web pages and other documents from your computer.

Software	Cost
YeoSoft Text to MP3 Speaker	$20
TextAloud	$30

Is it worth it? Do these programs offer enough services beyond the free Windows Narrator to justify their cost? Yes. First, Windows Narrator only reads screen names to help you navigate the interface—it does NOT read documents. The premium programs can also save audio files (of a text reading) so that you can listen to them later. If you want to listen to all of your emails while strolling around the neighborhood, you need to buy the other software.

Magnifiers

Magnifying software allows you to magnify all of your computer screen, sections of your computer screen, or localized areas beneath your mouse pointer. Again, Windows Vista features a magnifier and most web browsers include a magnifying feature, which increases font and image size for everything on a web page.

Here are a few more consumer magnifier products:

Software	Description	Cost
Windows Magnifier	Magnifies a portion of the screen into a separate window.	Free with Windows
SeeIt Magnifier	Magnifies the computer screen up to 32 times. Magnify the entire screen or a selected area.	$300

ZoomText Magnifier	Enlarges everything on your computer screen. This product boasts a clean text font appearance at all magnifying levels. You can optionally get the reader software, which will read the screen to you.	$200 on Amazon, with a list price of $350. With screen reader, cost is roughly $550.

Is it worth it? Some of these tools provide a much better interface than the Windows Magnifier. If you have vision challenges, then spending a few hundred dollars could make your computer experience more enjoyable.

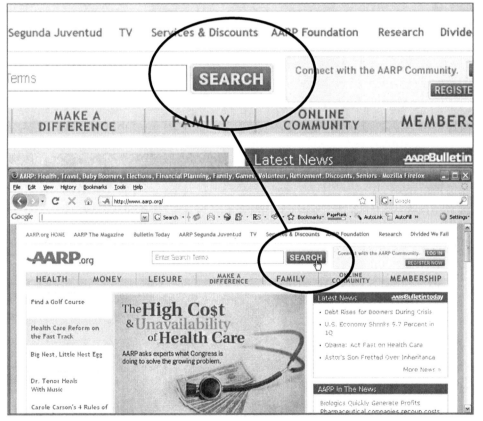

Magnifier feature in Windows XP. The area above your pointer (in this case, the circled pointing finger) is magnified above the window. This can be a little disorienting at first, but you'll get used to it.

Speech Recognition

Speech recognition is the opposite of Text to Speech. Rather than converting text to sound, speech recognition takes sound (your voice) and converts it to either text or computer commands. This can be an invaluable tool for computer users with severe arthritis or poor eyesight.

For example, you want to write a letter to your daughter thanking her for the latest subscription to Senior Sleuths of America. You sit down near your computer and speak a few commands to open a new Microsoft Word document. Then you simply speak the content of your letter, periodically speaking the command to save the document. You can then edit the document either through the keyboard or via voice commands. Finally, you issue the voice commands to print the document.

No speech recognition software is perfect. Although the best software out there (Dragon Naturally Speaking) boasts 99% accuracy, other online reviews put the actual number closer to 80%. That's still pretty good for no typing.

In a recent review of Nuance's Dragon Naturally Speaking software on the cnet.com website, Microsoft Vista speech recognition was mentioned as being about five years behind the Dragon technology. And because speech recognition is Nuance's bread and butter, it's a safe bet they'll stay ahead of Microsoft.

You're now probably waiting for the list of top speech recognition programs out there. It's a short list of one: Dragon Naturally Speaking 10 Preferred. This product is consistently ranked above all others, and the cost is a very reasonable $130 (reasonable for what you're getting). If you want to relieve stress on your hands and eyes, give some serious thought to this technology.

Task Simplification

New computer users can feel overwhelmed by the number of menus, buttons, and optional configuration settings in each and every computer screen. A few companies have created software to help these new users adjust to these overwhelming digital technologies.

One such company is Qualilife, the creators of the QualiWorld software platform. This platform supports a number of popular software applications that are simplified for easier access. This includes more accessible programs for surfing the Internet (QualiSURF), sending emails (QualiMAIL), writing documents (QualiWORD), making phone calls through the Internet connection (QualiPHONE), and many more.

The SeniorPC currently ships with some of these products. It's worth taking a look at the company's website to learn more about their offerings. Individual software programs range from $150 - $300. The entire suite (QualiWorld platform) is well over $1,000.

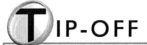

TIP-OFF

Other software offerings by QualiLife include: speech, webcam, TV, radio, DVD, chess, and cards. QualiLife also offers a very neat product called QualiEYE, which converts head or finger movements into screen actions. So you could, let's say, move your chin left and then the mouse pointer would also go left. It does this using a camera to track your motion. Pretty nifty!

Finding Reviews on Software

With thousands of software programs to choose from, how do you know that you're buying a high-quality product? Elementary, Dear Sleuth! Just read the reviews.

Here are three good online resources for researching software before buying:

✓ Software Review Websites

✓ Amazon.com

✓ Google

Software Review Websites

There are hundreds of websites that provide technology reviews. The trick is finding the good reviews rather than fake reviews written by the company manufacturing the product. The following two sites feature quality reviews with a good level of detail. Of course, they can't review each and every program out there, but if they do review the software you're interested in, the review will help you get a better idea of the software's strengths and weaknesses.

Proceed to one of the websites and type the name of the software in the search field at the top of the page. If the software is listed along with an "Editor's Review," then you're in luck! They have an in-depth review waiting to be read.

www.cnet.com

www.pcmag.com

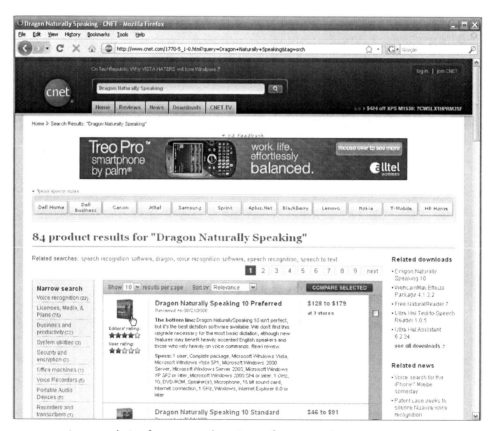

cnet.com is a good site for comprehensive software reviews.

Amazon.com (www.amazon.com)

Amazon features less formal customer reviews. Go to the amazon.com website, type the name of the software you are interested in, and scroll down the page to the Customer Reviews section. Although these aren't professional reviews, you can usually get a pretty good feel for a product by looking at the overall ranking (5 stars is best, 1 is worst).

If you're satisfied that the product looks good, you can scroll back up to the top of the page and purchase the product (i.e., Add to Shopping Cart).

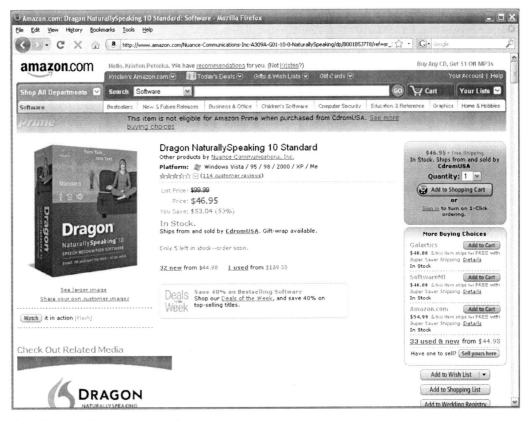

Scroll down the page to read user reviews on amazon.com.

Google (www.google.com)

Use Google (www.google.com), the world's most popular web search engine, to look for specific software reviews. Simply type the name of your software and the word "review," and click the **Search** button. Use quotations around the search parameters to focus your search—this searches for exact phrases and keeps you from getting two million unrelated results. For example, type **"Dragon Naturally Speaking" review**, and click **Search**.

You can then look through the search results for something that looks like an official review. Be careful not to depend too heavily on reviews posted on the product's website, unless you can verify that the review was performed independently by a reputable company.

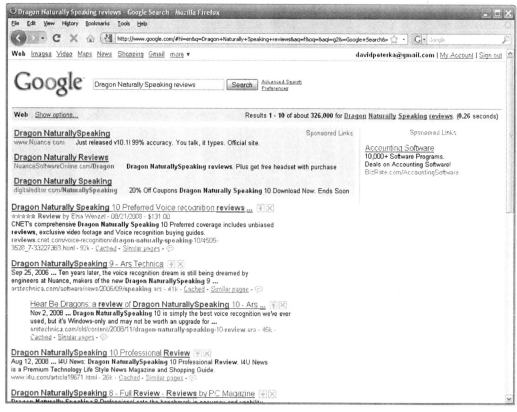

You can find anything using Google's search engine—including software reviews.

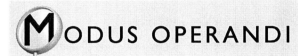MODUS OPERANDI

How to find a software review.

For this example, we'll locate a review on the speech recognition software Naturally Speaking using CNET.com.

To find the review on CNET.com:

1. Open a Web browser (like Internet Explorer).

2. Enter the following URL in the address bar at the top of the page: www.cnet.com

   The cnet web page opens.

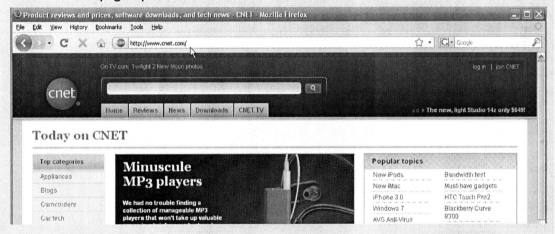

3. Type "Dragon Naturally Speaking" into the search box at the top of the page.

4. Press your **Enter** key.

   A list of results is displayed.

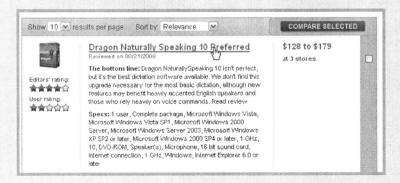

5. In the search results, click on the link to Dragon Naturally Speaking.

    The full review page will open. In this case, there is an Editor's review, so we're in luck! Read the detailed review and check out the links for where you can purchase the software.

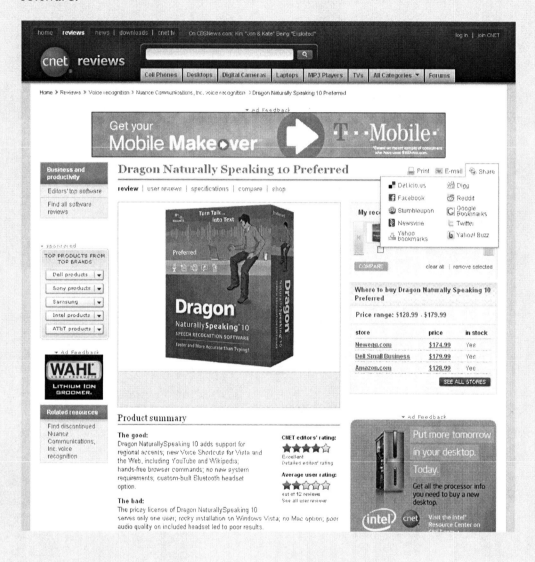

The Shift to Online Services

Many popular software applications are shifting to an online offering. This means that rather than installing the program onto your computer (by purchasing a CD or DVD and then copying all of the files onto your machine) you can simply go to a website with the same functionality as the installed software.

An example of this shift from computer-installed software to online service is TurboTax. A few years ago, you needed to install TurboTax on your computer. Now you can go to their website, enter your tax information, and submit your forms—all without installing a single piece of software onto your machine.

I mention this because you will often have the option of ordering an installation CD, downloading the installation files from the web, or using an online service. If you opt for an online service, then make sure to keep your receipt and any passwords they give you to access their online software. You'll need this information for upgrades and continued access to their site.

Remote Computer Help

Computers require routine maintenance and every so often they break. Maybe a single software application is no longer working. Maybe it takes ten minutes to open your email. For these types of minor performance problems, there's a nifty way to get help from your trusted friend or family member. You can let them control your computer from their computer, thus providing help from their own home.

This is particularly helpful if your personal technical support lives far away or if you just need some emergency help at odd hours (though I don't recommend calling family for tech support at 3AM—most things can wait until after morning coffee).

How do they work?

You need to install special Remote Access software onto your machine and (depending on the software you're using) onto the machine that will access your computer. Then the remote computer user (your kid or friend who used to work for NASA) uses the software to take control of your computer from their computer. They can search through your files, move your mouse, and perform maintenance and updates. They can do anything remotely that they could do if they were sitting at your actual computer.

This is really neat, but there is obviously room for abuse here. Make sure to only grant access to your computer to trusted people. Remember, they can scan your computer for private files (for example, financial information and passwords) so if your friend has evil tendencies, you might be in trouble.

Remember that you can also learn to service your own computer. There are a lot of online resources and books for performing maintenance on Windows and Macs. If this interests you, give it a try. If not, getting remote support from trusted family or friends could the way to go.

Here are a few popular software programs that provide remote computer access.

Software	Notes	Cost
Remote Desktop for Windows	This comes with some Windows machines, but there are a lot of operating system restrictions. For example, a Windows Vista computer can not connect to a Windows XP system. Also, you need to have the Professional version of Windows (XP or Vista) on the computer you intend to connect to. That means that you, the senior, would need to install the Professional version of Windows—which is almost certainly overkill.	Free with Windows XP Professional or Windows Vista Professional
GoToMyPC	This earned the pcmag.com Editor's Choice award. Access the remote computer from any modern Web browser.	$20/month (and up)
Laplink Everywhere	Similar features to GoToMyPC, but also features support for slower Internet connections (i.e., dial up). Also, the cost is half that of GoToMyPC.	$10/month
I'm InTouch	Similar to Laplink, but with slightly better full-control features.	$10/month

Software	Notes	Cost
LogMeIn Basic	FREE! You can have full remote control for FREE. Did I mention this is FREE? The only drawback is that you can't share files between the computers—something your support guru may want to do to fix a problem on your machine. You can work around this by telling the remote computer to email the files you want.	FREE

Here's my suggestion. I strongly recommend trying the free LogMeIn Basic before paying for one listed above. If you find yourself using the service all the time, then it might be worth paying for a slightly more robust program.

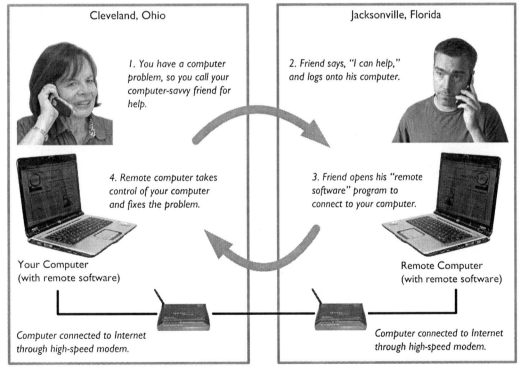

Remote computer setup.

Viruses and Security

Don't panic!

You might get a computer virus (a harmful computer program designed to wreak havoc on your computer). And someone might also illegally gain access to your computer. These things happen. But there are a few things you can do to 1) prevent these attacks, and 2) manage your data in such a way that you don't really care if you get attacked.

Antivirus Software

Antivirus software protects your computer from viruses and other harmful software referred to as malware. Antivirus software programs download regular updates from the Internet so they know which viruses to protect against.

If you are connected to the Internet (which you should be, because the Internet is fantastic), then you definitely need some form of antivirus software.

Here are three antivirus software suggestions from pcmag.com. CNET also has reviews for antivirus software programs, and Consumer Reports has an official ranking (available to subscribing members only).

Software	Notes	Cost
Norton Internet Security 2009	Receives good marks from most reviews. Many users complain that their online technical support is lousy. This is considered by many to be the best antivirus available.	$35
Kaspersky Internet Security 2009	Reviews note that the program is fast (which is great), but the interface is somewhat lacking (which is not great).	$35
Trend Micro Internet Security Pro 2009	Reviews mark the user experience better than Kapersky and on par with Norton. It costs a little more, but not much.	$45

Software	Notes	Cost
http://free.avg.com/	This is an open source antivirus for Windows. Although this free software is not as powerful as the above programs, it is FREE!	FREE!

Protecting Sensitive Data

If by some small chance a virus or hacker slips through your computer defenses, then they could gain access to all of the sensitive data on your machine. There is one foolproof method for keeping your sensitive data safe.

Do NOT put sensitive data on your machine!

A cyber thief can't steal your bank account number from your computer if you don't have your bank account number on your computer.

Just be careful.

I learned recently that my mother had created a Word document on her machine entitled "Passwords," where she listed all of her user IDs and passwords for her email account, bank accounts, and online brokerage. If this file were to fall into the wrong hands, mom's money could quickly slip from her hands.

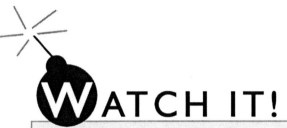

WATCH IT!

Do NOT save sensitive information on your computer in an unprotected file. Keep passwords and bank account information in your head or other safe location (like a safe). Computers can be broken into and your information stolen.

An alternate approach is to use a password management software to store multiple passwords and other sensitive data in a secure format. For example, use RoboForm (www.roboform.com) to store your bank login information. Next time you go to the bank's website, the password will be automatically populated for you in a secure way that is nearly impossible for hackers to monitor.

Try to avoid storing the following information on your computer:

✓ Bank account numbers.

✓ User name (or ID) and passwords for financial websites.

✓ User name and passwords for your email account.

✓ Passwords for any site. Pick something that you can remember and store it in your head.

✓ Social Security Number. This one can be tricky. For example, if you use TurboTax, then the forms store your social security number. After submitting your taxes, you should consider removing these files from your machine.

The Internet

Now that you know all about computers, the second stop on your Senior Technology investigation is the Internet.

The Internet has been around for over a decade, so there is an excellent chance that you have Internet access in your home. If you don't, I'm guessing that you soon will. The senior community represents the quickest growing segment on the Internet. According to SeniorNet, nearly 66% of Americans aged 50 to 64 use the Internet. Jupiter Research reports that Americans 50 years and older represent 33% of all US Internet use, making this segment the largest demographic on the Web. And over 70% of Baby Boomers have broadband Internet in their homes.

All of these numbers boil down to one cold hard fact. Seniors are online.

But how are they getting online? Which Internet sites provide the best services for seniors?

Great questions, Senior Sleuth. Let's go find some answers.

In this chapter you will investigate:

➤ What is the Internet? How does it work?

➤ Research Tools

➤ Websites for Seniors

➤ Online Shopping Sites

➤ How To Avoid Senior Scams

Background Check

What began as a small government project to share information between select research centers has exploded into a tool that has transformed modern life worldwide. The Internet has enabled new fantastical means of communication, commerce, and entertainment. And it all happened in the last 5 decades. Amazing!

Check out this high-level timeline to see a few major milestones in Internet technologies.

1955

1958
Funding approved by President Eisenhower for ARPA (Advanced Research Project Agency).

1969
ARPANET, the precursor to the Internet, developed by BBN. ARPANET created a communication link between universities and research centers. The first three nodes that formed the ARPANET were UCLA, Stanford, and the University of Utah.

1972
First basic email program created by BBN.

1978
TCP/IP protocol created. This is the modern protocol for the Internet, which specifies how data is sent between computers.

1980
Tim Berners-Lee creates the predecessor to the World Wide Web.

1983
Domain Name Systems (DNS) designed, thus establishing the .com, .edu, .gov, .mil, .org, .net, and .int nomenclature.

1984
"Cyberspace" term coined in William Gibson's "Neuromancer."

1985
First domain is registered. Symbolic.com.

1986
5000 host computers on ARPANET.

1989
100,000 host computers on ARPANET.

1990
ARPANET project ends. The modern World Wide Web is created by Tim Berners-Lee.

1993
Mosaic web browser created.

1994
Netscape founded. Microsoft buys technology to create a Web Browser for Windows 95.

1995
Sun Microsystems releases Java, a powerful programming language for the Internet.

1996
Browsers fight for market share. Netscape and Microsoft battle it out.

1999
Napster created, allowing peer-to-peer file sharing, creating problems for music and content producers.

2000
The Dot-Com bubble bursts. The majority of the Internet start-up businesses go out of business. Wikipedia.org launches.

2001
The start of the Internet marketing boom.

2005
YouTube.com video site launched.

2006
Approximately 100 million web sites online.

2007
1.2 billion people using the Internet worldwide.

2008
Google becomes the "most popular global brand."

2010

What is the Internet?

The Internet is a world-wide network of interconnected computers (hardware and software), which allow people to quickly share data. The Internet is a broad category of communication tools, which includes the World Wide Web (WWW, or simply the Web), email, instant messaging, and file-sharing applications. The Web refers specifically to documents and web pages connected through hyperlinks and URLs.

Does this distinction—Web versus the Internet—matter? Not really.

These two terms have practically become synonymous. For the rest of this book, we'll use the term Internet to refer generically to the broader mechanism that hosts the World Wide Web, email and instant messaging technologies.

Sure, fine. That's all nice, but how does it work?

All computers on the Internet share a common transfer protocol (a type of language), which enables them to send and receive information. Each computer on the Internet is also given an address (called an IP Address) so that other computers know where to send information and know where information originates. And sitting in between these computers are often powerful servers, which can index information and act as routing devices between individual computer addresses.

A reasonable analogy would be the US Postal Service. You have a package you want to send to your cousin Charlie. You write his address on the package, include your own return address and then drop it in the mail. The package proceeds through one or more post offices, following the USPS mail handling procedures, until it finally reaches Charlie.

The Internet is similar, but instead of sending a package from one address to another, you are sending a packet of data. And in between the two addresses (your computer and the target computer), your data may be routed through a server rather than the post office. And rather than the USPS procedures, the Internet uses a standardized set of communication protocols.

Not that any of this really matters, unless you're planning on going back to school to study Computer Science and Engineering. For our purposes, the Internet allows us to access information and data which is stored on another computer. The reason that this is such a powerful technology is because there are a lot of computers out there, each of which can store volumes of information. The bottom line is this—lots of data is at our fingertips.

Accessing the Internet

Any reasonably modern computer is equipped to access the Internet. The four most common approaches are:

✓ **Dial-up.** Use a modem (inside your computer) to dial a phone number that links you into an Internet server.

✓ **High Speed Internet through DSL or Cable.** Use a special high-speed modem to send and receive data through your existing phone or cable lines.

✓ **Wireless.** Access the Internet through over-the-air signals.

✓ **Satellite.** Send and receive Internet data through—you guessed it—a satellite.

Dial-Up

Dial-up Internet connections are slow—achieving a maximum data transfer rate of 56 kilobits per second, which equates to loading an average web page in around 7 seconds. This is the least expensive method of Internet connection, but no matter the cost, it's not worth it. Better to pay more and get a fast connection. Trust me on this one.

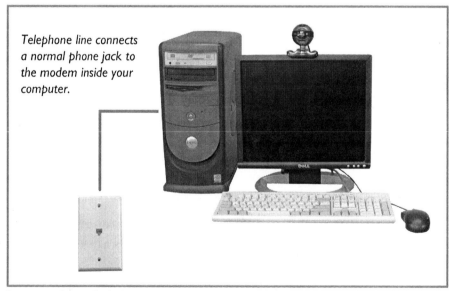

Telephone line connects a normal phone jack to the modem inside your computer.

Internet through dial-up connection.

High-Speed (Broadband)

High-speed Internet is fast—thus the name. In fact, it is up to 50 times faster than dial up. Special high-speed modems (external to your computer) receive data through your existing phone or cable wires. You then plug your computer into the high-speed modem. Unfortunately, high-speed Internet is not available everywhere. If you live in off-the-beaten-track farm country or at the top of a mountain, high-speed may not have reached you (yet). If, however, you live in an area that does offer high-speed connections, think seriously about getting it.

Installation is relatively straight forward and once it's up and running, you can forget it's there. Unlike dial-up where you have to dial in to a server every time you want to check your email, high-speed Internet is always connected. Just turn your computer on and you are on the Internet.

It will cost you around $20/month or more (depending on your package). It's absolutely worth every penny.

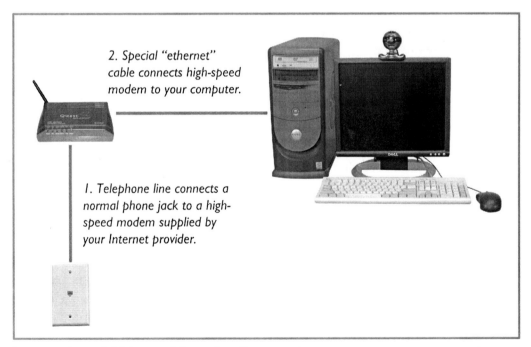

2. Special "ethernet" cable connects high-speed modem to your computer.

1. Telephone line connects a normal phone jack to a high-speed modem supplied by your Internet provider.

Internet through high-speed (broadband) connection.

Wireless

Most laptops are now equipped with wireless network cards, which can connect to the Internet without any wires. In order for this to work, you need to be within a hundred feet or so of a wireless router, and that router needs to allow you to access it, but this isn't as restrictive as it sounds. Almost every coffee shop and thousands of other restaurants and bars are providing free wireless access to customers.

If you have wireless capabilities on your laptop, then you still need to get some sort of Internet service in your home. Again, I strongly recommend a high-speed connection. With the correct configuration, your laptop will be able to connect to the Internet from anywhere in your home.

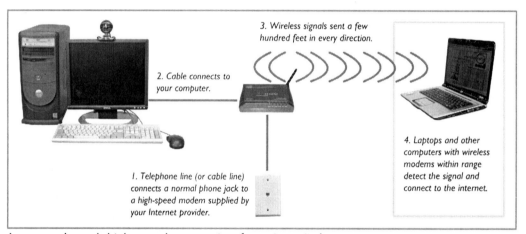

Internet through high-speed connection featuring wireless access.

Satellite

If high-speed Internet is not available at your home, you should consider Satellite before settling for dial-up. Satellite Internet sends and receives data through—you guessed it—a satellite. As long as you have a clear view of the Southern sky, you can get an Internet connection. Satellite is much faster than dial-up, but slower than a DSL or cable-based high-speed connection. It is, however, the most expensive Internet service.

Mobile Internet

Planning on spending the next few years exploring the country in your RV? If so, you can stay connected to the Internet. More and more RV campgrounds are offering wireless Internet. Just park, turn on your wireless-enabled laptop, and connect to the Internet through the campground's provider.

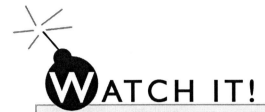

WATCH IT!

Make sure to read the instructions and warning on the wireless modem (usually comes with your high-speed Internet). They will instruct you on how to secure your wireless connection from the bad guys.

If that solution isn't good enough for you—you need Internet for each and every stop—then you can purchase a portable satellite dish made specifically for RVs. Simply point the RV-mounted satellite in the right direction and get reasonably fast Internet no matter where you are. Of course, the dishes are several thousands of dollars, and there is a monthly fee (around $80/month), but you can't beat the convenience.

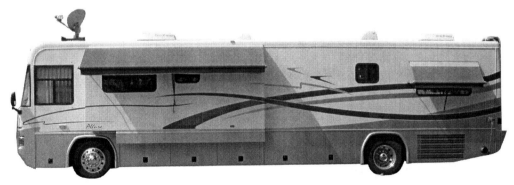

Satellite dish on top of RV = Internet anywhere you can drive.

JUST THE FACTS

Comparing Internet Connections.

Take a look at the speeds, costs, and availability of the different Internet connection types.

Internet Connection	Data Download	Approx. $/month	Availability
Dial Up	56 kbps	$5	Anywhere that has access to a telephone line.
Broadband High Speed (DSL or Cable)	128 kbps to 20 Mbps	$20 to $60	Most major metropolitan areas and surrounding suburbs get access through either their phone or cable provider. Check your provider to see if they have high-speed Internet for you.
Satellite	1.0 Mbps and up	$60 and up	Available anywhere with line-of-sight access to the southern sky.

Researching on the Internet

The Internet has put more information at our fingertips than we could ever read in one, two, or even a thousand human lifetimes. The key to successfully navigating the Internet is knowing how to find the trustworthy information that you want to find.

The two best ways to locate information on the Internet are:

✓ Search Engines

✓ Trusted content websites

Search Engines

Internet search engines are Web pages that allow you to search for other Web pages containing a word or phrase. Let's say that I wanted to find information on US Census bureau statistics on senior citizens. I would open up my favorite search engine, and type the words US Census bureau statistics senior citizens. I would then click the **Search** button on the page and instantly receive 52,000 search results. The pages with content that best match my search criteria are listed first.

Search engines will usually be your first stop on the Internet. In fact, you might want to make one of them your browser's Home Page (the page that first opens when you open the browser).

Here's a quick look at the most popular search engines.

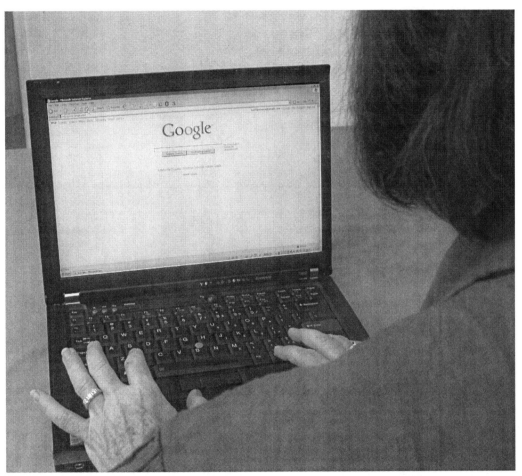

Seniors can search for ANYTHING using one of the popular search engines, like Google.

Google

Google is the most popular web search engine in the world. And for good reason—it's fantastic! The page is simple and arguably serves up the best search results. It uses a proprietary results ranking program that ensures you always get good results.

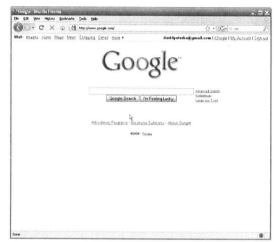

All search engine websites include advertising—paid adverts for companies with products or services that in some way relate to your search. Google does a nice job of making these inconspicuous—blending them into the side of the page so you barely notice them. If, however, you are looking for paid ads, then the results are actually quite helpful.

Google home page.

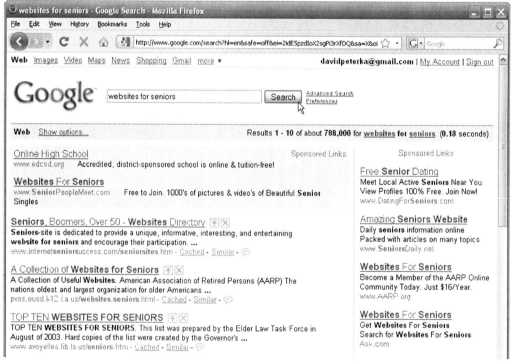

Google search results page is also clean and simple. The ads (Sponsored Links) are on the right side of the page.

Yahoo!

Yahoo! also gives you good search results, but their default home page is cluttered with multiple categories, news headlines, and big annoying graphical advertisements. You can customize your Yahoo home page to be simpler (or more complex), but that takes clicking around a different configuration page. This may be worth the effort if you always want to see the same types of information when you first log onto the Internet. For example, you can choose to display top headlines from CNN, the local weather, and some statistics on your favorite sports team when you open up your Web browser. You just need to configure your Yahoo home page to do this. It's pretty easy, actually.

Note that the other search engines also provide this type of configurable home page, where you can display clippings of information from multiple sources. Google and Yahoo take opposite approaches. Google starts with a clean, blank search page that you can add to. Yahoo starts with a messy, cluttered page that you can subtract from or modify.

Just one more thing... Remember that the less content you need to load, the

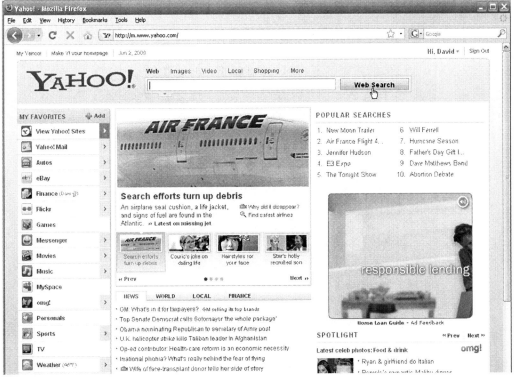

Yahoo! home page.

quicker the page will come up. So if you find yourself starting every Internet session with a quick search and don't care about all of the extra information, then simplify your home page.

MSN (now Bing)

MSN's popular search engine was given a face-lift in 2009 and renamed Bing. If you perform a web search from www.msn.com, you will be forwarded to the Bing interface. Microsoft seems to have taken a page from the Google handbook and simplified their interface. The result is a much cleaner look.

The search engine results are also fine. Really, it's hard to quantify which search engine actually gives you the best results. They all seem to do pretty well. The only obvious difference between the search engines is appearance. Google (and now Bing) are simple and uncluttered, and Yahoo! is busy. This is not a judgment. You may prefer to have all of the information displayed for you. If you do, then Yahoo! is probably the search engine for you.

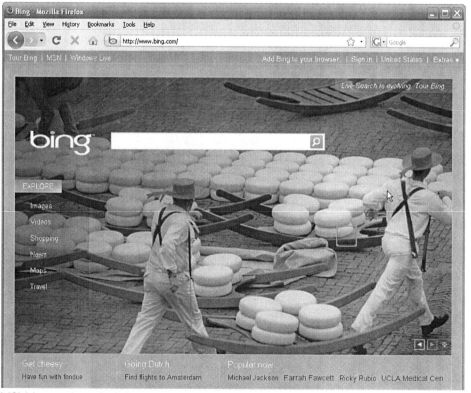

MSN has re-branded their search tool as bing.

MODUS OPERANDI

How to set your Home Page in Internet Explorer

The Home Page is the first website that opens when you start your Internet Browser. Here's how you set your home page for the Internet Explorer browser (the browser that comes installed on all Microsoft Windows machines):

1. Open (or launch) Internet Explorer.

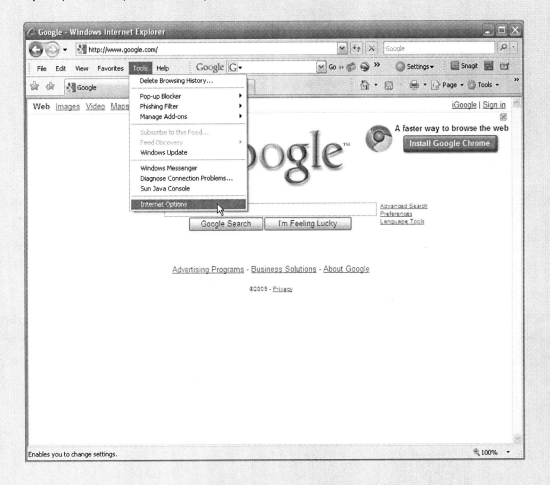

2. From the menus at the top of the page, select **Tools > Internet Options.**
   The Internet Option window opens.

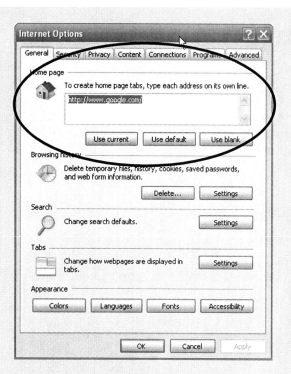

3. In the Home Page field, enter the Web address (also called the URL) of the site that you want to make your home page.

   For this example, I set the Google home page (`www.google.com`) as my home page.

4. Click **OK** to save the setting and close the Internet Options window.

Now whenever I open the Internet Explorer browser, it will display the Google home page. This is a great starting page for two reasons: 1.) I usually want to search for things when I get online, and Google is a great search engine; and 2.) Google doesn't include a lot of graphics and so loads really quickly. But that's just me. Feel free to set your home page to any page on the World Wide Web.

Advanced Web Searches

Because you are a Senior Sleuth, you might be curious about advanced search features. These tricks help you refine your searches to ensure the best results each and every time.

All search engines include an "Advanced Search" feature, which will return only those results which meet all of your advanced requirements, such as:

✓ ALL of the search words must be included (in any order) in the result

✓ The exact phrase must be included in the result

✓ Any of the words must be included in the result (example: car or boat)

✓ Exclusion: the results can NOT include any pages with one or more specific words

Each of these advanced search parameters can be accessed from a separate Advanced Search screen. Google provides a link to their Advanced Search from their main page. Yahoo and Bing only provide the link after you've performed your initial search.

You can also access these advanced features on the main search page by typing your search terms in a specific way. For example, if you want to search for a specific phrase, place the phrase inside quotation marks. Here is the syntax for the most common advanced search features.

Advanced Feature	Syntax for Search Field	Example
Include Exact phrase	"search term"	"where is my flying car"
Include ANY words	Word OR Word	flying car OR jetpack
Exclude word	Word −Exclusion	Flying car −blimp

Most of the search engines do a nice job of prioritizing their results and will often give you great results from a standard search. Google claims that their own employees use the advanced features less than 5% of the time. You probably won't need these, but if you do, here they are.

Reliable Research Sites

The amount of free information on the Internet is staggering and powerful and wondrous. The problem you quickly run into is trust. What information can you believe? Yes, there is a lot of great information out there, but for every trustworthy fact there are twenty bits of misinformation. Whether the bad information is put there on purpose (to confound your Senior Sleuthing) or inadvertently by someone who just got it wrong, you need to be able to filter the good from the bad.

The following websites are—for the most part—great resources for your senior sleuthing.

Research Website	Description
Wikipedia www.wikipedia.org	Wikipedia is a collaborative online encyclopedia. Anyone can create and edit articles. This results in thousands and thousands of articles on a huge range of topics.
	This site is a great first stop for any investigation. It usually provides a fantastic topic overview and list of additional resources.
	You do, however, need to take the content with a grain of salt. Although the material is usually quite good, the site is not officially fact-checked. So bad information does sneak in.
	If you encounter misinformation or have additional information regarding a topic of interest, create a Wikipedia account and then update the page. The more knowledgeable the people that create and edit Wikipedia content, the better the site becomes, following the old adage (and here I'm paraphrasing), "several thousand minds are better than one."

Research Website	Description
How Stuff Works www.howstuffworks.com	How Stuff Works is a professionally developed site that provides free information on—not surprisingly—how stuff works. Always wanted to know how the moving pictures get onto your television screen? Just type "Television" into the How Stuff Works search field and away you go. This site does an excellent job of presenting technical information to the novice. By the end of an article, you will understand how a particular piece of technology works.
Encyclopedia Britannica www.britannica.com	Premium (pay) site. If you must have hard, confirmed facts, you might want to subscribe to the online version of Encyclopedia Britannica. For $70/year you can access all of the content in the official print edition plus additional videos and other supplemental content.
WebMD www.webmd.com	WebMD provides trusted medical information. Curious about that new throbbing pain in your big toe? Search on WebMD to get a better idea of the cause and possible treatment. The WebMD people stress that this is an information-only site and is NOT replacing your doctor. Doctors are needed for definitive diagnoses and treatment plans. Use WebMD as a way to inform yourself (and to keep your doctor honest). The more you know, the better you can advocate for your own health.

Research Website	Description
Google Scholar	Google Scholar provides an easy way to search for scholarly abstracts and articles. In fact, you use a search page similar to the normal Google search. Some of the scholarly papers are available for free, although you'll have to pay to read many of them. If you're working on a serious academic venture and need the latest research, then this is a powerful tool.
Yahoo Answers answers.yahoo.com	Do you have a specific question that you need answered, but can't seem to find any coverage using a normal web search? If so, try Yahoo Answers. First, search through their site to see if someone else has already asked your question. If they have, then check out the answer. If not, post your question and wait for someone to answer it. The answers usually come pretty quickly. And they are often very good. You can ask any question—from technology to fashion to travel. Remember that these answers are coming from relatively anonymous sources, so you should use the information cautiously—especially if the information can result in injury or destruction of property (yours or someone else's).
Financial Research Sites	There are dozens of good websites that provide financial news and analyses, and tools for managing personal finances. If you want to research a particular stock price or want to calculate how much money you can safely spend in retirement, then these sites are worth a look. Here's a list of the three most popular financial sites: ✓ Yahoo! Finances (finance.yahoo.com) ✓ AOL Money & Finance (money.aol.com) ✓ MSN Money (money.msn.com)

Research Website	Description
Travel Research Sites	There are hundreds of websites serving the travel market. You can now research your destination, find hotels, book flights, and read reviews on everything from food to accommodations before you purchase your ticket. We investigate these travel websites later in this book. See Chapter 7 Travel and Transport.
Weather www.weather.com	Planning a trip up the coast or a walk around the block? Better make sure that the weather is going to cooperate. You can now get an extended 10-day forecast from weather.com. You can also research weather trends and averages, and check out other helpful weather facts like the daily pollen count or air quality. Really, I don't know how we lived without this information before.

Websites for the Senior Community

Where there is a need (or an audience) for information or services, there is a website. Actually, there are usually thousands of websites. As the fastest growing segment of the Internet, Seniors provide an obvious market for online entrepreneurs and large companies looking to get their message out to their audience.

Here is a tiny sampling of available websites that serve the senior community. This list is meant to whet your appetite. If you're looking for

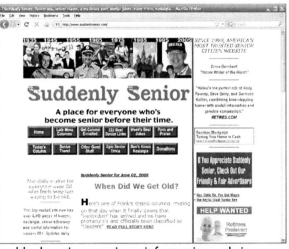

suddenlysenior.com is an informative website.

something specific, just use your favorite search engine to find it.

Informational Websites for Seniors

There are too many senior websites to list them all in this book. So, I'll list a few of my favorites, which cover a broad range of topics. These sites all include links to other websites of interest to seniors. So you can start at one of these pages and follow link after link after link after link to other interesting senior websites.

AARP.org

The website for American Association of Retired Persons (AARP) is a great resource—even for non-members. It provides relevant and insightful articles on topics related to health, money, leisure, family, and technology for the senior community. It also includes AARP surveys and research. Did I mention this is all for free?

AARP.org also provides a list of their favorite senior websites at `www.aarp.org/internetresources`.

seniorjournal.com

Seniorjournal.com is an online senior daily news site. This site contains good articles on varied senior topics including health and fitness, government, entertainment, the web, elder care, and money. The articles are produced by the Senior Journal staff.

The site itself is cluttered with advertisements, but the articles are good. It's worth a visit.

Seniorjournal.com also includes a list of websites of interest to seniors. Check out the following link to see their recommendations: `www.seniorjournal.com/seniorlinks.htm`.

suddenlysenior.com

The Suddenly Senior website features "humor, nostalgia, senior advocacy and useful information for seniors 50+." The site is somewhat graphically challenged, but the content is good and entertaining. It's also another good starting point for senior reading. Check out its list of 222 senior links at `www.suddenlysenior.com/links.shtml`.

assistivetech.net

This site devoted to assistive technologies is a great place to research the latest technologies for people with special needs. This is a wiki-type site (like the popular website wikipedia.org), so it can be updated by anyone. It is therefore likely to list products as soon as they become available—sometimes even as soon as they are conceived. Remember to treat this information as a starting point only. Wiki content can never be 100% trusted.

usa.gov

The US government offers a senior section on their website. The following page provides a slew of links to senior information, laws, and services. Topics include caregiver resources, consumer protection, health, lists of federal and state agencies for seniors, senior housing, money, retirement, and travel.

`www.usa.gov/Topics/Seniors.shtml`

Administration on Aging (aoa.gov)

The Administration on Aging is another US government resource for aging Americans. This site provides information and services for seniors, their families, and professional caregivers. Topics include community support services, nutrition, preventive health, caregiver support, and senior rights.

Online Dating Websites

Yes, seniors date. And the Internet is making it easier to find partners with similar interests, compatible personalities, and reasonable proximity. For many people, online dating still has a stigma associated with it, but that negative attitude is changing. In just the last year, I've met a dozen charming (and happy) couples that met through an online dating service.

Seniors can take advantage of online dating sites specifically for seniors. They all offer similar features including searching based on common parameters like age, sex, and interests. They all also charge a monthly fee, which can be cancelled as soon as you find your match.

TIP-OFF

Almost all of the following sites provide a limited access "free" membership, but in order to really benefit from the site, you'll have to upgrade to the premium membership.

Website	Fees*
singlesover50.com	$49.95 for 3 months, $69.95 for 6 months, and $99.95 for 12 months. Membership prices are posted in their Help section.
Seniormatch.com	$29.95 for 1 month; $59.95 for 3 months; $95.95 for six months; $143.95 for 12 months.
Seniorfriendfinder.com	Offers silver and gold memberships. Gold provides more photos and places your profile higher in other people's searches (which sounds a little like cheating). The site doesn't post its prices up front (you have to first create an account), which seems a little sneaky.

* Note that many of these sites will automatically renew your membership unless you actively cancel it. Unfortunately, this practice is common among all types of online memberships sites.

Travel Websites

There are hundreds of websites serving the senior travel market. You can now research your destination, find hotels, book flights, and read reviews on everything from food to accommodations before you purchase your ticket.

We'll investigate these travel websites in Chapter 7 Travel and Transport.

Communication

The Internet provides countless methods of keeping in touch online, including email, social networking sites, photo sharing sites, and blogs. We'll investigate these communication tools in more detail in Chapter 6 Communication.

Medical Information

You can also find dozens of websites for researching medical information and managing your health records. We'll investigate these websites in Chapter 4 Health and Medication.

Online Shopping

Online shopping, sometimes referred to as e-commerce, has revolutionized how we buy everything from groceries to cars. We can now research products, compare prices, and purchase new and used goods from the comfort of our living room. Of course, sometimes you'll still want to go to a store to feel the fabric or smell the candle before buying, but for many items, shopping online saves you the trip to the store and usually snatches up a lower price.

Consider the following different types of online shopping options.

Amazon.com

Amazon.com is America's largest online retailer. Although Amazon started out in 1995 selling exclusively books, it quickly moved into the market of music, videos, consumer electronics, sporting goods, home appliances, and more. Basically, they sell everything.

Nearly half of the Amazon sales are through what they refer to as Amazon Associates. These are individuals who sell products through the Amazon website, granting a percentage of their sale proceeds to Amazon. This results in a huge and diverse product offering and allows everyone to sell (almost) anything through Amazon.

Amazon also features customer reviews of products, so you can get a sense of quality before you purchase.

To get started, just type in the product you want to purchase in the Amazon search field at the top of the page and click **Go**.

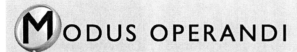ODUS OPERANDI

How to Buy a Digital Camera on Amazon.com

Amazon.com provides a nice shopping experience where you can compare prices and read user reviews.

To buy a digital camera on Amazon.com:

1. Open a Web browser (like Internet Explorer).

2. Enter `www.amazon.com` in the Web address field and click **Enter** on your keyboard to go to the website.

3. In the Search field, enter "digital camera" and press Enter on your keyboard.

   Several pages of search results are returned.

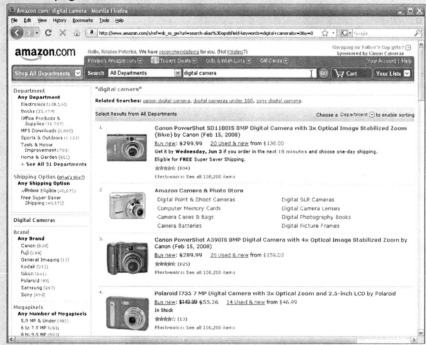

4. Skim the list to find a camera that fits your budget and use.

   Pay attention to the user ratings (number of stars). More stars means a better rating.

5. Click the name of the product.

   The product detail page opens.

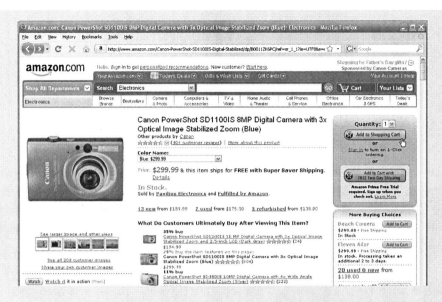

6. Read the Web page including the Product Details, Product Description, and Customer Reviews to ensure that this product meets your needs.

7. At the top-right of the page, click the **Add to Shopping Cart** button.

   TIP: You can optionally browse through the "used & new" section (linked on the right) to find a great deal on a used product from a private seller.

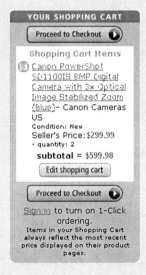

8. Click the **Proceed to Checkout** button on the next page.

9. Enter your email address and specify whether you are a new or returning customer. If you are a new customer, you'll be asked to create an account. If you are an existing

customer, enter your password to complete the transaction.

10. Enter your billing information (e.g., credit card information and billing and shipping address), and follow the prompts to complete the transaction.

Amazon is a secure site, so it is safe to enter your credit card information.

Ebay

Ebay is an online shopping website where users bid on new and used items in an auction style. The winner of the auction gets to buy the object—often at a huge discount over retail price. Sellers often offer a **Buy It Now** option, where the buyer can close the auction by agreeing to the seller's stated price.

Ebay features seller reviews and rankings so that you can feel confident that you'll actually get the product you paid for. Be cautious when purchasing from a seller with very few reviews or negative reviews—these can indicate fraudulent sellers or just plain bad customer service. It's better to pay a little more to a good seller and actually get your product than to pay less to a bad seller.

Buyer beware, but don't let this discourage you from trying it out. I have bought over a hundred Ebay items over the last several years and have always received what I paid for. Just check the seller's reviews and you should be OK.

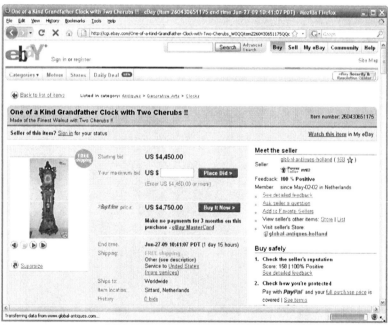

Listing page on ebay.

MODUS OPERANDI

How to Buy a Digital Camera on Ebay.com

Ebay is a great place to go to buy used material. You can often get great deals on used goods, but you need to be careful not to get swindled. Read the seller reviews before you bid on their products and you should be fine.

Also note that Ebay is an auction site where you can place "bids" on products. The winning bidder gets the product. Some items include a "Buy it Now" option, where you can end the bidding period by agreeing to a specified price.

To buy a digital camera on Ebay.com:

1. Open a Web browser (like Internet Explorer).

2. Enter www.ebay.com in the Web address field and click **Enter** to go to the website.

3. On the main page, click the **Register** button to create an Ebay account. Fill in the fields and follow the on-screen instructions to complete your registration.

   You will need an account in order to complete any transaction on Ebay.

4. In the Search field, enter digital camera and press **Enter**.

   Thousands of search results are returned. Rather than page through all of the items, we'll filter the results. Note that you can also search for a specific model name—Canon Powershot, for example—to focus the results.

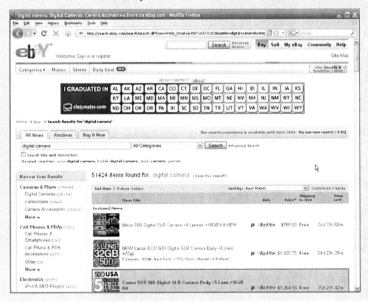

5. Under Narrow Your Results on the left side of the page, click the `Digital Cameras` link.

   This filters out everything but cameras from the search `results`. It also opens the "Digital Camera Finder," which allows you to narrow your results further.

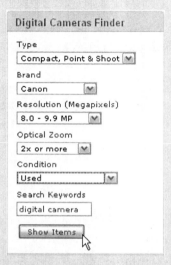

6. Narrow the results by selecting the values from the drop down list. For this example, we select Type (Compact, Point & Shoot), Brand (Canon), Resolution (8.0 - 9.9 MP), Condition (Used).

7. Under the Digital Camera Finder, click **Show Items**.

   A much smaller list of items is displayed.

8. Skim the results to find a camera that fits your budget and use.

   Be careful here—these are used items. Make sure they are fully functional and include any plugs or batteries required for operation.

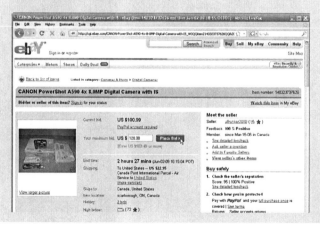

9. Click the name of the product to view the product details page.

10. Review the following information:

    ✛ Seller Feedback—you want to see something very close to 100%.

    ✛ Shipping and Handling price—a low selling price with an outrageous shipping price is not a good deal.

    ✛ Payment method—many sellers accept credit cards, but some only accept payment through an online payment service called Paypal. You may need to create a Paypal account (www.paypal.com) to complete the transaction.

11. If the item includes a "Buy It Now" option, you can optionally click the **Buy It Now** button and proceed through checkout.

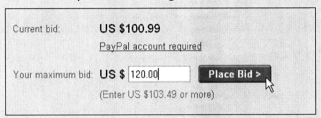

12. Otherwise, enter your bid in the Your maximum bid field and click **Place Bid**.

    Ebay will only bid up to as much as your maximum on your behalf. If you hold the maximum bid, Ebay will stop bidding at the next highest bid. For example, let's say your maximum bid is $100 and the next highest is $80. Ebay will stop bidding at something like $82 (an amount just above the next highest).

    At this point you are winning the bid. As long as nobody else comes along and out bids you, you will get your camera.

13. Follow the seller instructions for completing the transaction and sending payment.

Craigslist.org

Craigslist is a popular community-based website where you can search for or post classified items for sale, personals, job opportunities, and other services. Craigslist offers a great opportunity for shoppers. If someone in your metro area has what you want, you can often buy it from them for a great price. Additionally, you save on shipping charges because you can simply go pick it up. This also reduces the opportunity for fraud—you don't hand over the cash until they hand over the goods.

Craigslist.org is available in most metro areas in the US and in several other large cities internationally.

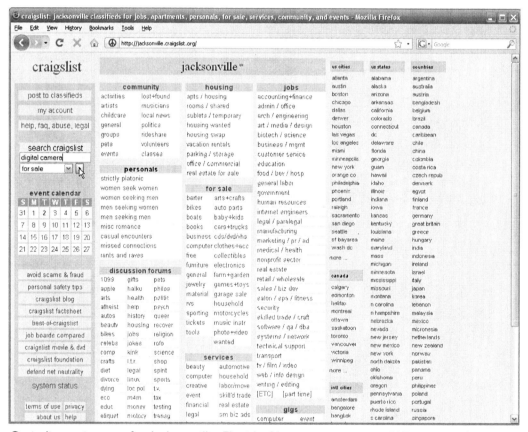

Craigslist main page for Jacksonville, Florida. Almost every major U.S. metropolitan area has a similar Craigslist page.

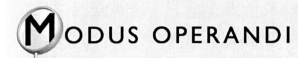 Modus Operandi

How to Buy a Digital Camera on Craigslist.com

Craigslist.com lets you buy mostly used goods from people in your local area.

To buy a digital camera on Craigslist.com.

1. Open a Web browser (like Internet Explorer).

2. Enter `www.craigslist.com` in the Web address field and click **Enter** on your keyboard to go to the website.

   The first time you use craigslist you will need to navigate to the listing for your city or metro area. For this example, we'll navigate to Jacksonville, Florida.

3. Click the link to `Florida` and then click the link to `Jacksonville` on the next page.

4. The Jacksonville craigslist page opens.

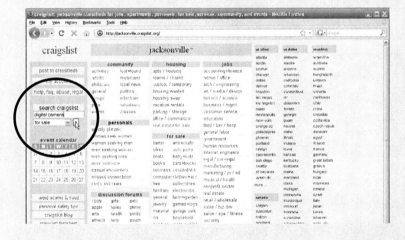

5. In the search craigslist field on the left, enter `digital camera` and click **Enter.**

   Depending on what you are searching for, hundreds of search results can be returned. You may need to filter the results down a bit more. Note that you can search for a specific model name—Canon Powershot, for example—to focus the results.

   You can also enter a minimum and maximum price on the results page to find only cameras within your budget.

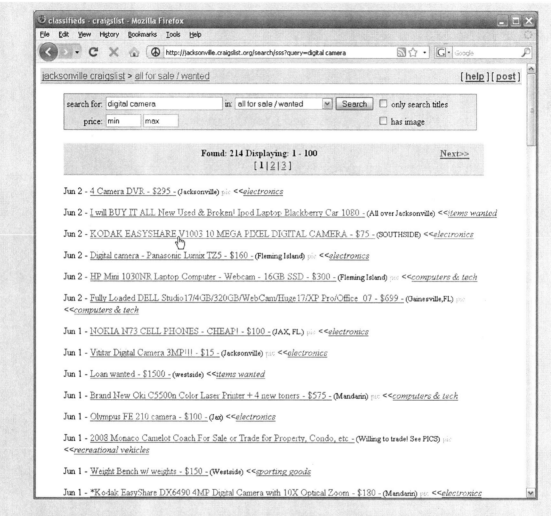

6. Click through the results to see the full listings of cameras that fit your budget.

    Be careful here—these are used items. Make sure they are fully functional and include any plugs or batteries required for operation.

7. When you find a camera you like, look at the bottom of the page for the seller's contact information.

    The seller will provide either an email address or a phone number.

8. Contact the seller to see if the item is still available. If it is, you can negotiate a time and place to pick up (and pay for the item).

Remember that the real power of Craigslist is the local listing. This means you can actually see what you are getting when you go pick it up (before you hand over any money). If the seller demands payment before you see the item, just walk away. It's probably a scammer.

"Bot" Shops

There are a number of shopping websites that gather information from other shopping sites and display information on the product and stores where the products are being sold. These "bot" (short, I presume, for robot) websites provide a quick way to check the availability of a product and get a sense of the price range at different stores. Once you find the product, you can click on a merchant's link to buy the product from that online store.

Bot websites will usually give the seller a rating and include information on their shipping costs. If Seller X has the best product price, but he charges a twenty dollars for shipping, then you might be better off going with Seller Y, who offers a slightly higher price but free shipping.

Note that these sites don't check ALL other shopping websites. For example, Ebay will not be listed. If you're willing to buy a used product, you can usually get great deals through Amazon, Ebay or Craigslist instead of using the "bot" shop.

Two comparable "bot" shopping sites are www.shopzilla.com and www.pricegrabber.com.

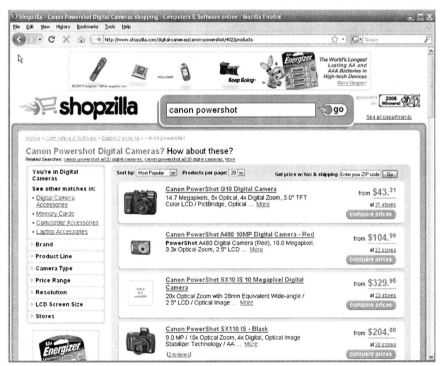

Shopzilla search results for a product.

Overstock.com

Overstock.com is a bargain website. They purchase excess stock from other retailers and then sell them through their site. Yes, they sell these items at a slight markup for them, but the prices are still a great bargain for you.

Because overstock.com never really knows what's going to be next month's overstocked items, their product offerings are fluid. Sometimes there's really great stuff on their site, sometimes it's junk.

If you love buying things BECAUSE they are on sale, then you might love overstock.com.

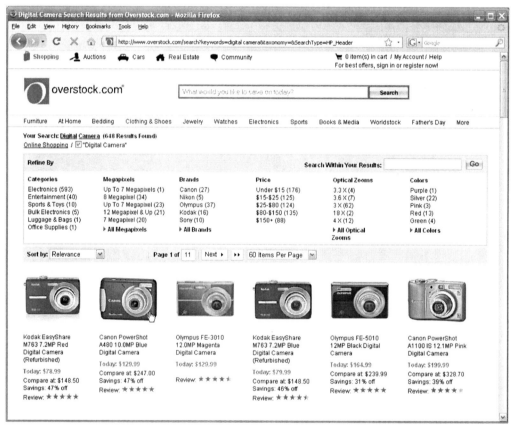

Overstock search results for a digital camera.

[Name of Retail Store].com

Almost every chain retail store has an associated online store. For example, you can buy anything offered in the Sears store through their website www.sears.com. You won't necessarily get the best deals on these sites, but you can generally expect good reliable service. If you are a loyal customer and don't mind spending a little extra money on your products, use your favorite bricks-and-mortar stores' websites to make your online purchases.

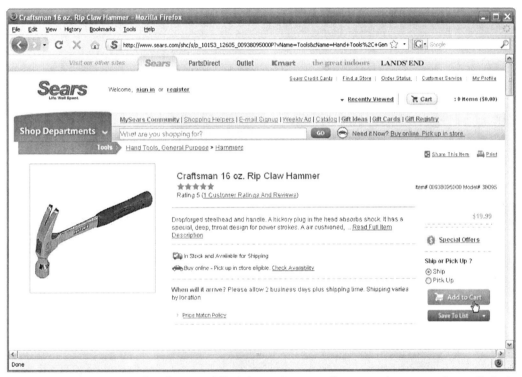

sears.com is just one of a thousand "bricks-and-mortar" stores that now also sell their merchandise through a website.

Avoiding Internet Scams

The FBI reported that Internet fraud comprised 44% of all FBI complaints in 2007. These included check fraud, undelivered merchandise, credit card fraud, and confidence frauds. The FBI provides good tips for avoiding Internet scams on their Internet Fraud webpage at `www.fbi.gov/majcases/fraud/internetschemes.htm`.

Here are some FBI suggestions for avoiding Internet Fraud.

Fraud	How to Avoid
Internet Auction Fraud	Read the seller's feedback and check the Better Business Bureau (if the seller is a business). Never give your Social Security Number to a seller.
Non-Delivery	Make sure the seller is a reputable company by checking reviews and the Better Business Bureau. Don't respond to unsolicited special offers that you receive in your email. Make sure the company has a real address (not just a post office) and a working email address.
Credit Card Fraud	Only give your credit card number through "secure" sites of reputable companies. Check the Better Business Bureau and other online reviews of the vendor. Remember that you can usually dispute credit card charges if someone uses your card inappropriately.
Investment Fraud	Research ALL investment opportunities before putting money into them. Remember that a flashy website can be created in a few hours and does not mean the company that created it is legitimate. "If it sounds too good to be true, it probably is." (This sentiment is repeated on almost every fraud prevention website. If everyone says it, it must be true.)

Fraud	How to Avoid
"Nigerian Letter Scam"	This common scam features a letter (or email) from a foreign government, claiming that they need to offload a large sum of money into your account. For the convenience, they claim that you can keep a portion of the money.

Ha!

It is simply not true. If you receive an email with something similar to this, delete it. Don't respond. Just delete it.

No matter what you do, DO NOT give anyone your bank account information in an email. (In fact, you really shouldn't give your bank account information to anyone except a banker or finance officer.) |

Other Senior Scams

The FBI also provides information for Senior-specific scams. They explain why seniors are often a target for criminals and provide tips for avoiding the most common scams. The scams include healthcare fraud, counterfeit prescription drugs, funeral fraud, fake anti-aging products, and telemarketing schemes.

See the following Web page for more information.

www.fbi.gov/majcases/fraud/seniorsfam.htm

TIP-OFF

You can also check out information on senior scams and other senior alerts at http://seniorjournal. com/Alerts.htm. This website provides timely alerts on scams and safety notices impacting the senior community.

5 Quick Tips for Using the Internet

✓ **Buyer beware.** If an online deal sounds too good to be true, it probably is. That said, there are some really, really exceptional deals out there. If the deal is posted on a reputable website, then maybe it is true.

✓ **Use trusted websites.** If you want to buy a sink, it's probably safer to order it from Homedepot.com than to order it from GetCheapSinksBeforeItsTooLate.com. Remember that you can usually find reviews of websites by typing "[Name of Website] review" into your favorite search engine. If nobody has reviewed the website, then it might be a scam.

✓ **Never share usernames and passwords.** Would you give a stranger the combination to your wall safe? Usernames and passwords can be used to access such things as bank accounts and other sensitive information. Keep these private and safe. Optionally, you can buy a password management software to safely store your sensitive data.

✓ **Don't click links in emails from people you don't know.** Clicking these links can download viruses to your computer and mark you on a "sucker" list. If you don't trust the sender, don't click the link.

✓ **The Almighty Restart.** Sometimes your Internet connection will just stop working. This could be a problem with your local phone or cable line or could just be a hiccup in your high-speed modem. If you have a problem accessing any web pages, then restart your modem (turn it off and then back on). More often than not this will get the data flowing again. If this doesn't fix the problem, restart your computer. If neither of these work, then the problem might be with your Internet provider. In this case, grab a good book, pour yourself a glass of wine and wait. It'll be back soon enough.

Health and Medication

Everyone gets sick. That's just the way our bodies work. As we get older, more chronic conditions of aging creep into our medical lexicon. High blood pressure? Ulcer? Arthritis? Sigh. We get more aches and pains, which require more pills, which require more medical interventions. Before you know it, you're taking ten pills a day for five different conditions.

Keeping track of all of your doctor visits, medical history, and medications can be mind numbing—even if you are relatively healthy. It gets exponentially more complicated when you add one or two or more medical conditions to your personal health story.

Fear not, Senior Sleuth, for as I'm sure you have already deduced, there are some nifty technologies that help track and manage the complexities of caring for the human body.

In this chapter you will investigate:

➤ Tools for managing and distributing medication

➤ Medical devices for the home

➤ Online tools for home health management

➤ Interesting medical research

Background Check

We're living longer. This is great, but it also opens up the opportunity for contracting illnesses later in life. The longer we live, the more opportunities our bodies have to break. Fortunately, doctors and researchers have gotten really good at diagnosing and fixing a bunch of these problems.

If you were born in 1900 (which you probably were not), your life expectancy was roughly 50 years. Yikes. If, however, you were born in the 50's and 60's then your life expectancy jumps up to around 70 years. This is better, but I'm still shooting for a spry 140. Wouldn't that be cool?

Why are we living longer today than ever before?

Another excellent question, Senior Sleuth. The answer is simple: technology.

The 20th Century saw a boom in healthcare and drug technologies, including:

✓ Insulin, a drug for managing the deadly diabetes, was developed in the early 1920's.

✓ Penicillin, an antibiotic used to treat bacterial infections, was discovered in 1928.

✓ Mass vaccinations were initiated to prevent deaths from such diseases as yellow fever, measles, and mumps.

✓ Advances in medical imaging, computers, and materials allow doctors to identify problems early and then address them surgically with pinpoint accuracy.

TIP-OFF

Medical Imaging and Surgical Techniques

Without delving too deeply into this topic, let's just say that today's medical technologies are amazing! Using modern technology, doctors can:

✓ Detect cancer early with enhanced medical imaging

✓ Perform heart surgery without cracking open your chest

✓ Replace a hip or knee as an outpatient procedure

The bottom line is if something hurts, tell your doctor. There may be a new therapy or technology that can fix whatever pains you. And if there isn't one available today, your doctor might know of some promising research coming down the line.

Managing Medication

Forgetting things is normal. It can also be dangerous—especially when it comes to medication. There's a reason your doctor tells you to take, say, your blood pressure pills before each meal and heart meds once daily. It's because he knows (or at least has an extremely educated guess) how much help your body needs to function properly. Too many or too few drugs or drugs taken at the wrong times could lead to a trip to the emergency room.

Your doctor prescribes how much medication to take and when to take it. All you have to do is follow the directions. Unfortunately, things come up and we forget. If only there were tools to help us remember to take our meds and ensure we take the right ones.

Well, Senior Sleuth, there are such tools. Check out the following technologies for managing your medication.

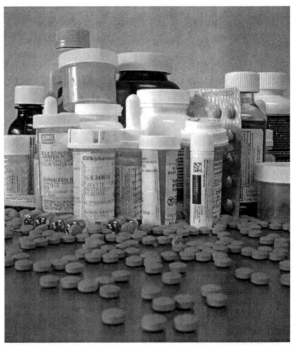

As we get older, we might need to take more and more pills.

Medication Reminders

Sometimes an alarm clock just doesn't cut it. This is especially true when you need to be reminded of things several times a day and may not be anywhere near your nightstand. This is why the technology gods created medication reminders.

Medication reminders come in the following flavors:

✓ Watches with multiple alarms

✓ Pill boxes with integrated reminder alarms

✓ Phone reminder services

Reminder Watches

These suped-up wristwatches get the job done. Most models feature several alarms and a few of the fancier models include visual indicators of which medicine you should take with the alarm. The more high-tech features the watch has, the more it will cost you.

Here are a few available reminder watches. There are dozens more models available, so check out the web (and read reviews) before settling on a model. This probably goes without saying, but if you need to remember to take medication five times a day, then a watch with only four programmable alarms won't cut it. Also, you might want to allow some room for expansion. You never can tell when your doctor will add two or ten more pills to your daily regiment.

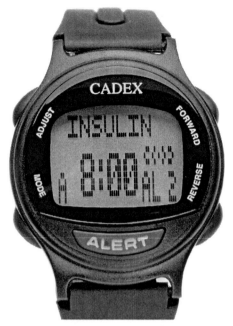

Courtesy e-pill® Medication Reminders
www.epill.com
1-800-549-0095

Watch	Features	Cost*
CADEX Medication Reminder Watch	12 daily alarms; reminder messages (program the name of your medication); medical ID setting to display any serious health conditions to emergency medical staff.	$80
e-pill MeDose Vibrating 6 Alarm Watch	6 daily alarms; vibration or sound alarm. Note: There is a non-digital (i.e. with hands) model available for $200. Pretty expensive, but it looks sharp!	$100
HealthWatch 100	8 daily alarms; reminder medication display; records your pill-taking history; interfaces with PC for programming your schedule and storing data.	$250

* Prices taken from www.epill.com, a good site for medical gadgets.

Pill Boxes with Reminders

Since you'll most likely keep your pills in a pill box, it kind of makes sense that your pill box would incorporate some sort of reminder technology. What good is a beeping watch when your pills are three counties away? These electronic reminder pill boxes cost a little more than the simple plastic pill organizers, but they also beep or vibrate! The prices are modest—cheaper, in fact, than the reminder watches—and they work.

Here's a small sample of available pill boxes with built-in reminders.

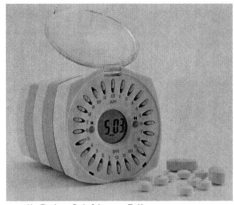

e-pill Cube 24 Alarm Pill
Courtesy e-pill® Medication Reminders
www.epill.com
1-800-549-0095

Pill Box	Features	Cost
e-pill POCKET Pill Box	Size: Compact Reminder: beep or vibration Number of daily alarms: 4 Capacity: 4 medication compartments (holds several pills in each)	$40
e-pill Cube 24 Alarm Pill	Size: Compact Reminder: beep only Number of daily alarms: 4 Capacity: 30 small tablets in each box (up to 4 boxes) Features a missed pill indicator.	$30
e-pill Multi-Alarm PLUS Pill Timer Pillbox	Size: Moderate (fit into large pocket or bag) Reminder: beep only (long duration) Number of daily alarms: 37 Capacity: 7 compartments (holds several pills in each) Features a missed pill indicator.	$50

CLUE

I realize that the above section feels like an advertisement for e-pill products. It's not, I promise! They happen to have a lot of well-advertised products. Don't take my word for it, though. Perform your own online investigation. Search for "pill box timer" and see what pops up. A lot of the results will be e-pill products.

Phone Reminder Services

Phone medication reminders used to only work when you were at home, but now, assuming you have a cell phone, you can receive friendly medication reminders at pre-arranged times no matter where you are.

Here's a sample of phone reminder services. Both services feature automatic notifications sent to contact list if you don't answer the call.

Call Service	Features	Cost
Angel Telecare Inc.	Reminder: phone call with recorded reminder Number of daily calls: Up to 12 (price listed is for 3 calls/day; price goes up for more calls) www.angeltelecare.com	$30/month
Database System Corp. CARE Call Reassurance	Reminder: phone call with recorded reminder Number of daily calls: No specified limit. www.medication-reminders.com	$25/month (monthly cost goes down if you commit to several months)

Recommendation: With other affordable reminder technologies available, the phone service loses some of its appeal. Why have someone else remind you when you can program your watch or pillbox to remind you?

You can easily spend $360 each year with these services. So you could purchase several of the other reminder products—say a watch and a pill box timer—for the same money as one year of phone calls. To me this is a no-brainer. I prefer the gadgets. And it's not like you're gaining companionship from the call service. It's not a real person calling you—it's a recording. If, however, you are gadget averse, reminder calls could be just what the doctor ordered.

Medication Dispensers

What if you don't just want to be notified that it's time to take your medication? What if you want your pill organizer to actually spit out the appropriate pills for you at the right time of the day? Then you want a high-tech medication dispenser.

Because these devices only dispense the correct medication at the correct times of the day, there is little chance of medication error. You can't take pills early, and if you take them late, notifications will be sent to your family or caregiver. Some of these devices also come with handy locks so there is no way that rotten Billy Jenkins down the block can break into your pills.

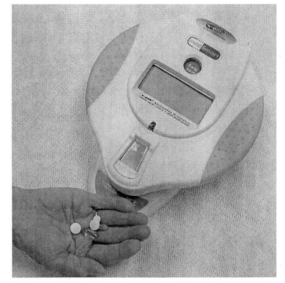

These automated devices are really helpful to those seniors who need extra help with medication management—for example, seniors with early stages of Alzheimer's or other cognitive problems that could lead to missed pills or accidental overdose.

Without a doubt, these fancy dispensers are expensive. But when you compare them to the cost of a phone reminder service,

e-pill Monitored Automatic Pill Dispenser
Courtesy e-pill® Medication Reminders
www.epill.com
1-800-549-0095

they are quite reasonable—even the most expensive device pays for itself in less than 3 years. And when you compare the cost of these devices against the cost of an emergency room visit for medication-related emergencies, then they seem outright cheap.

If you have a complex daily medication routine where deviation could result in an emergency, then you may want to check these out.

Just one more thing... Although each of these devices boasts "easy setup," you still need to load all of your medicine and set the timers in order to get the full benefit of the "automatic" dispenser.

Dispenser	Features	Cost
e-pill Automatic Pill Dispenser	Includes Reminder: Yes (28 per day) Number of Daily Dispenses: 28 Lockable: Yes Handheld: Yes Notable Features: When alarm goes off, the pill compartment rotates to let the pills dispense. Alarm shuts off when you turn the device upside down to retrieve the pills.	$395
MedSmart Locked Automatic Medication Pill Dispenser	Includes Reminder: Yes (6 per day); Beep and blinking light. Number of Daily Dispenses: 6 (comes with 2 trays with 29 compartments each, so you could go several weeks between refills) Lockable: Yes Handheld: Yes Notable Features: When alarm goes off, the pill compartment rotates to let the pills dispense. Alarm shuts off when you turn the device upside down to retrieve the pills.	$595

Dispenser	Features	Cost
Philips Medication Dispenser: MD2	Includes Reminder: Yes (6 per day); Voice, text and blinking light. Number of Daily Dispenses: 6 cups/day (holds 60 cups); 3-4 weeks between refills Lockable: Yes Handheld: No (about the size of a coffee pot) Notable Features: Sends alert to caregiver if meds not taken on time or if medication is running low.	$895
CompuMed Automatic Pill Dispenser	Includes Reminder: Yes (4 per day); Alarm and text. Number of Daily Dispenses: 4; 1 week between refills Lockable: Yes (they boast "tamperproof") Handheld: No (about the size of a coffee pot) Notable Features: Text message can include medication instructions	$895

Future Medication Managers

The next generation of pill reminder and dispenser products is in the works. Accenture, a global consulting company, has developed one such high-tech prototype. They call it the Online Medicine Cabinet.

This prototype features cameras and face-recognition software to identify a person and then uses its internal computer to identify your medicine and distribute appropriately. The cabinet would also monitor blood pressure and heart rate and then send that information over the Internet to your doctor.

This is the technological equivalent to the magic mirror. You stand in front of it and it tells you what you need to know. Are your vitals out of whack with your medical history? You'll be prompted to set up an appointment with your doctor through the cabinet's interface. Missed a prescribed medication? The cabinet will tell you and then tell you when and how to take the missed medicine.

It's all very neat. Look for another wave of these types of devices to show up on the shelves in the next five to ten years.

See www.accenture.com for more information on their online medicine cabinet.

Medical Devices for the Home

You don't have to go to the hospital to stay on top of your health. By keeping your eye on a few key vitals you can detect health issues early. If something stands out, you can then contact your doctor.

Here are a few health monitoring gadgets that have become fairly common in the home.

Blood Pressure Monitors

Blood pressure monitors come in all shapes and sizes and include different levels of automation. These can be tabletop devices or can be portable machines that you can wear on your wrist. You strap it on, push a button, and it automatically takes a reading.

There are hundreds of products available—all relatively inexpensive. You can get a quality machine for well under $100.

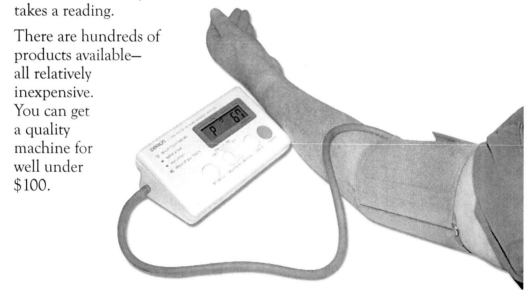

Wrap the strap around your arm, push the button, and wait for your the automatic blood pressure reading.

Heart Rate Monitors

Heart rate monitors have been popularized by runners and exercise enthusiasts. By monitoring their heart rate while exercising, these athletes can ensure that their heart is beating at the correct rate for, say, optimal fat burning.

Seniors can benefit from these devices in the same way—they can monitor their heart rates for optimal health. If you're exercising, then you'll want to make sure your heart rate is within a certain (doctor prescribed) range. If your heart rate is too low, you won't get optimal aerobic results. If it's too high, then you're risking injury.

Heart rate monitors come in two designs—both of which typically incorporate standard watch features, such as clock and stopwatch.

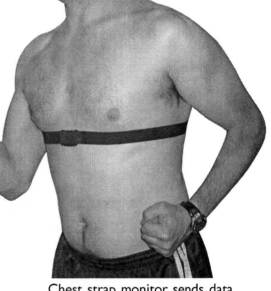

✓ **Monitor with chest strap.** Comfortable strap around the chest detects electrical heart impulses and then sends that information wirelessly to the paired wristwatch. These are the most accurate monitors.

Chest strap monitor sends data to the paired wristwatch.

✓ **Pulse monitor without chest strap.** Detects a pulse—usually by requiring you to place a few fingers on probes. These are less accurate, but don't require a chest strap.

The most basic models will only display the heart rate. More advanced (and more expensive) models will provide a host of other cool features: a link to your computer for logging your exercise, audible alarms to let you know when you are in and out of

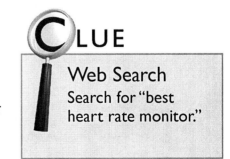

CLUE

Web Search
Search for "best heart rate monitor."

your optimal heart range zone, and pre-programmed exercise routines.

Prices range from around $25 for the most basic model to $200 for the most advanced models. There are a lot of great options that fall between these two price extremes.

Blood Glucose Monitors

If you are diabetic or borderline diabetic then you need one of these devices. They are small, inexpensive, fast, and only require a little blood for each test. Simply prick your finger, put a little blood on the tester strip, and place the strip into the machine. Your results can come back in as little as 10 seconds.

Costs range from around $20 to $150, with many options in between. Note that you'll need to also buy extra testing strips no matter which device you get. These can be pricey.

Make sure to read reviews before buying. There is a wide quality variation (how accurate the measurements are) between the devices.

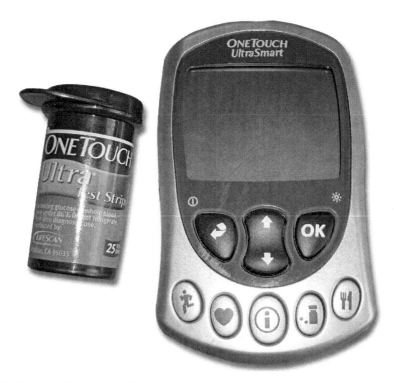

Prick your finger, swab blood onto the test strip, and insert the strip into the electronic monitor. You'll get your blood sugar reading within a minute. Pretty neat.

Home Defibrillators

There are a few medical devices previously only found in hospitals that have made their way into the consumer market. The defibrillator is one such device. These consumer-model defibrillators are light-weight and fully automated. They instruct you on where to put the electrodes, and then operate only when appropriate (i.e. the patient is in cardiac arrest).

Ranging from $1000 to $2000 for a consumer model, these devices are typically purchased by community recreation and sport centers rather than for the home. But if you have a heart condition and an extra thousand dollars lying around, you might want one of these things close by.

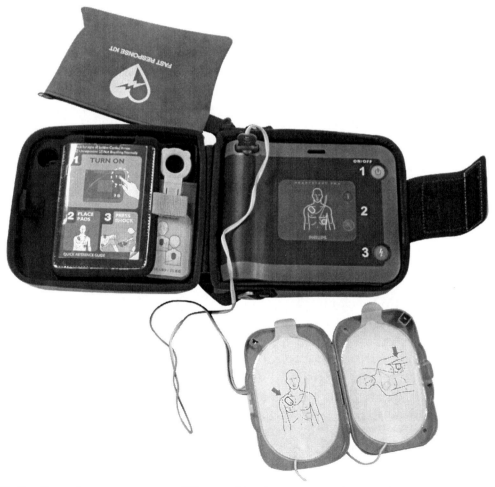

Defibrillator for your very own! The machine instructs you how to attach the pads and then only activates if it detects cardiac arrest.

Online Health Management

Complex prescriptions, future doctor appointments, visitation history, weight loss goals, immunization schedules, x-rays, MRI results, family medical histories...

The list goes on and on.

What is this list, you ask?

It's everything you need to know in order to stay on top of your health. Sure, your doctor may have some of this information in one of his file folders, but you probably don't have it. What if you want to change doctors? What if (and I hope this doesn't happen) there is an emergency and you need to be rushed to the ER? Then you need quick access to your medical history—including all prescriptions you are currently taking.

Luckily, there are some major players developing systems to help you manage your personal medical history. These systems store and manage medical data (history and medication) and then can share that information with your physician over the Internet. Of course, your doctor needs to be willing to also use one of these systems in order to realize the full benefits, but more and more doctors are signing up. It saves both the patient and doctor's time and leads to better care through better patient information.

Let's investigate two industry giants who have ventured into this market: Microsoft and Google.

Microsoft HealthVaultTM

Microsoft HealthVault is a platform for managing your personal health. What do I mean by platform? Think of a platform as the foundation and basic electrical scheme for your house. Other builders and companies can then develop products for your house—toasters, dishwashers, TVs, and telephones. Microsoft HealthVault is the foundation that supports other health-related gadgets and software. Microsoft develops and publishes standards and software so that other companies can build products according to those standards and become a part of the overall solution.

What does Microsoft HealthVault do?

HealthVault provides a Web interface where you can:

✓ Consolidate health information—including medical histories and current prescriptions—for all members of your family

✓ Share your health information with doctors

✓ Analyze your health data

HealthVault's main appeal is that it helps you simplify all of your medical records by storing them in a central location.

Because HealthVault has created a platform, other companies can develop products to interface with it. For example, there are HealthVault-certified scales that will automatically upload your weight to the computer. This can help you track your fitness over time. HealthVault-certified devices include:

✓ Weight scales

✓ Heart rate monitors

✓ Blood glucose monitors

These devices feature automatic (or really easy) data uploads to the HealthVault.

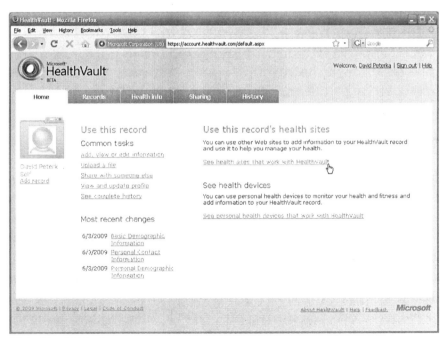

Main HealthVault page.

JUST THE FACTS

Microsoft HealthVault

How do you use it?

Create a free online account at www.healthvault.com. Purchase optional devices. Start managing your health.

How much does it cost?

Creating a HealthVault account is free, but almost everything else costs money. This includes downloading your medical history from your doctor. And don't forget that each gadget you want to integrate (for monitoring weight, heart, and blood sugar) also costs money.

You can enter your medical history by hand for free, but this could take a long time. Prices are reasonable and the products are all pretty good. The main HealthVault page includes links to supported software and devices. You'll have to visit each site to get their prices and detailed product descriptions.

Will my doctor be able to access my records?

Yes. Sharing your medical history with your doctor is a free service offered through the registeR4Health software. Your doctor also needs to subscribe to this service in order to see your records.

Google Health

Google Health is another platform for managing your health records in a central location. Like Microsoft HealthVault, Google Health allows you to integrate with other health software applications to import and share medical records. Similar to HealthVault applications, you need to pay to use many of the Google applications.

As of this printing, Google Health did not advertise or link to any approved medical monitoring devices (such as blood pressure, heart rate, and blood glucose monitors). On the flip side, Google seems to have a slightly more usable interface for entering personal information.

Visit www.google.com/health for more information.

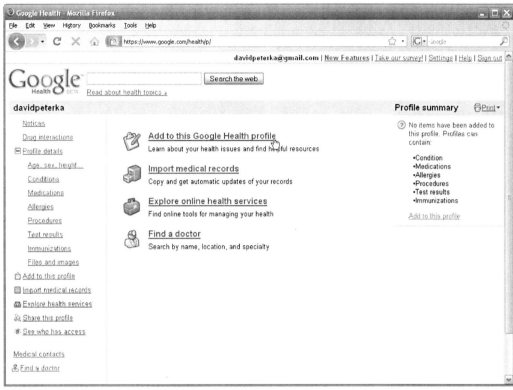

Google Health main page is clean and easy-to-use. Just what you expect from Google.

Microsoft HealthVault or Google Health?

At a glance, Microsoft HealthVault appears to offer more technological services and device integration. But both applications are positioned to make an aggressive play on the market. Google will most likely favor an open-source integration strategy, which could allow many more products to easily integrate with its platform. Microsoft seems to have a slight head start in the integration aspect, already offering several dozen integrated devices.

If you are going to integrate with one or more monitoring devices, you probably want to go with Microsoft. Otherwise, either platform will serve you well.

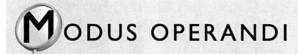ODUS OPERANDI

How to create a Microsoft HealthVault Account

Create a Microsoft HealthVault account to start managing your family's health records. Here's how to do it:

1. Open a Web browser (like Internet Explorer).

2. Enter `www.healthvault.com` in the Web address field and click **Enter** to go to the website.

   The first time you use HealthVault you will be asked to select whether you are an individual or healthcare representative.

3. Click the link for "individual" to proceed to the main HealthVault page.

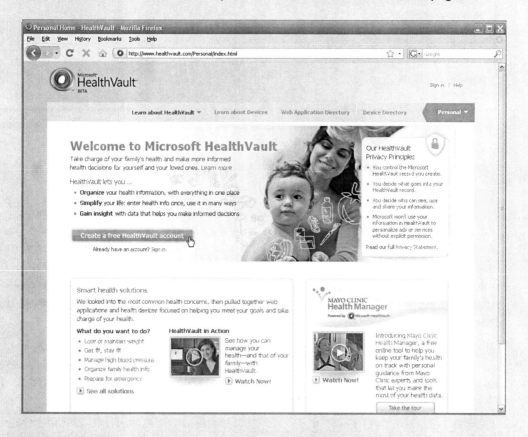

4. Click the **Create a free HealthVault account** button.

5. On the next page, enter your email address and click **Continue**.

   Note that you'll need a Windows Live ID. If you don't have one, then the Web page will lead you through the steps in creating one. In the following steps, I will proceed using my Yahoo! email address.

6. Create your Windows Live ID by entering information in the page and clicking the **I Accept** button.

7. On the next page, enter your personal information (such as name and address) and other required information.

8. Select the checkbox that says "I accept the terms and conditions..."

9. Click the **Create account** button.

   Your Microsoft HealthVault page opens.

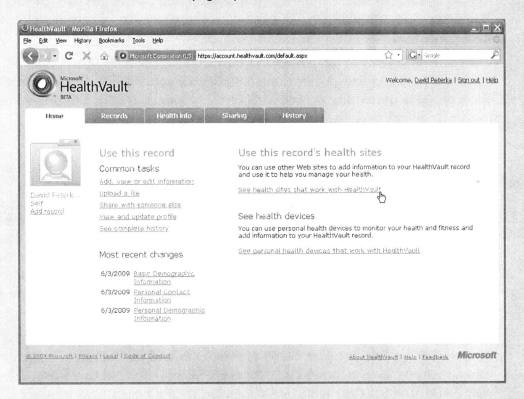

And you are done! Click through the links and tabs on your HealthVault page to add services and manage your health records.

TIP: Click the `See health sites that work with HealthVault` link to find services that will allow you to import your medical records from your doctor.

Medical Research and New Technologies

The last century has seen monumental improvements in digital imaging, drug therapies, medical monitoring devices and surgical techniques. Medical technology has been sprinting along. And it just keeps on going.

Here are a few interesting areas of medical research and technology that could re-revolutionize modern medicine.

Gene Therapy

Gene therapy is a method for treating genetic disorders. One future application of gene therapy could include manipulating cancer-causing genes to stop building proteins incorrectly, thus stopping cancer growths. New genes—the ones that fix or replace the defective genes—will likely be delivered via a controlled virus into the target body area.

Gene therapy is still in its infancy. So far human trials have been limited (with some ending badly), but there have been signs of hope. Recent trials show progress in treating people with certain types of genetic blindness, lung cancer (in mice), and deafness (in guinea pigs).

Scientists are getting closer to making this a consumer reality.

Embryonic Stem Cell Research

Embryonic stem cells have the ability to turn into any type of cell. This could be a great advancement in treatments of physical trauma and certain diseases! Let's say that you are showing off your juggling skills by flipping around three razor sharp knives. A gust of wind blows one of the knives off course and it chops off your finger, which then falls down a drainpipe into the sewer and is never seen again. Ouch!

Future (distant future) stem cell therapies could offer some help. Some day doctors may be able to take a batch of stem cells and instruct them to grow into bone cells, skin cells, and all other cells you might find in a finger. Then they could reattach the digit to your hand in time for your next juggling performance.

This type of therapy is still decades away, but there are some stem cell replacement therapies being used today to treat burn victims and people with blood disorders.

Brain Interface

Scientists and engineers are making progress in the realm of brain interface—creating a way to use signals from the brain to control a computer or other external machine. In fact, scientists have already implanted a chip into a monkey that allowed the monkey to move a robot just by thinking about it. Pretty cool.

This has obvious applications for amputees or people with limited mobility. Imagine controlling prosthetics or full exoskeletons with simple thoughts. The bionic man doesn't seem so exotic anymore.

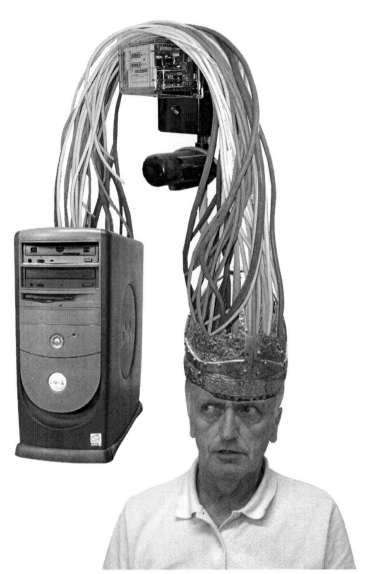

The fashion of the future? "Artist" rendering of electrode helmet for detecting brain waves, which can be converted into computer commands.

Independent Living

Independence.

It's not something that we're going to give up without a fight.

You've lived in your house for the last 50 years—provided shelter for 3 kids, 4 dogs, 7 hamsters, and 1 huge boa constrictor named Alfred. You know which rooms are coolest in the summer and warmest in the winter, which lamp throws the best light for reading, how many boxes of cereal fit in your cabinet. This is where you are most comfortable. This is where you want to stay.

But as we get older, staying in our home can get tricky. That table of knickknacks slowly shifts from a display of cherished memories to a tripping hazard. Your bathtub stops being a place of relaxing refuge and becomes the most dangerous area in your home. And you can all but write off the upstairs.

It's not that our homes get more dangerous—it's that the consequences of even minor stumbles increase exponentially. We all stub our toe and trip over things throughout our lives. But as we get older, our bones break a little easier and we heal a little more slowly. If we fall, there's a good chance that we'll need help.

Geez! What's with the gloom and doom?

You're right. You probably won't fall. You probably won't need someone's help. You can probably stay in your home for another 40 years without incident.

But that doesn't mean you couldn't benefit from one of the following "aging-in-place" technologies.

Let's investigate!

➢ **Task Simplification Technologies**

- ✦ Mailboxes
- ✦ Automation
- ✦ Door Knobs
- ✦ Hearing Aids
- ✦ Robots!

➢ **Home Monitoring Technologies**

- ✦ Monitoring Falls
- ✦ Monitoring Activity
- ✦ Monitoring Congnition
- ✦ Visual Monitoring

Task Simplification

As our bodies age, they slow down a bit and get a little unsteady. Activities that were once elementary slowly transform into significant challenges. For example, grasping and turning a door handle can be a problem for someone with severe arthritis. A walk to the mailbox—once a delightful excuse to get outside—can become a trip fraught with danger.

Rather than sit in your armchair all day, paralyzed by fear of daily living, you can use technology to keep yourself active. Here are a few technologies that can help simplify some every-day tasks.

Mailbox Alerts

If the weather is nice, then nothing is more pleasant than walking to your mailbox several times a day to see what the friendly postman has brought. Get outside. Enjoy the sweet smell of roses!

Imagine, though, your driveway is covered by a solid sheet of wintry ice. In this case, you should probably minimize the number of trips to the mailbox. Why risk falling—especially if the mail has not yet arrived?

Technology to the rescue again!

Now you install a small wireless device in your mailbox that will detect when the mail arrives and will notify you in the house. These products are easy to install and relatively inexpensive, ranging from $50 to $100.

Remember that mailboxes are still vulnerable to crazy bat-wielding teenagers, so you probably don't want to invest too much money into your mailbox technology.

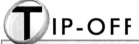

TIP-OFF

Junk Mail!
You'll never stop junk mail altogether, but you can significantly reduce the amount you receive. Online services such as Tonic's Mailstopper can reduce your junk mail (catalogs and other ads) by around 90%. It costs $20 per year, but it cuts down on irritating clutter and saves some trees in the process.

See `mailstopper.tonic.com` for details.

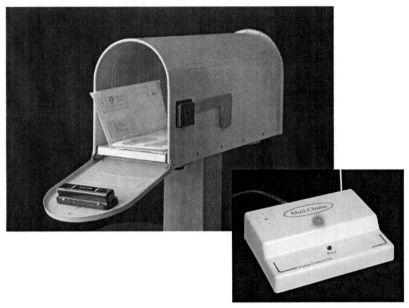

The Hanna Mail Chime alerts you when your mailbox opens.

Home Automation

Home automation can cut down on your energy consumption and can increase your home's safety. Motion-sensors turn on lights when you enter a room—preventing stumbles as you walk through the dark AND saving on electricity. Advanced thermostats keep the temperature comfortable during the day and cooler at night while you are safely beneath your blankets.

Additionally, you can install safety automation on burners and stoves to help you avoid burning down your house (an activity which I strongly recommend avoiding).

Home automation technology usually requires installation by

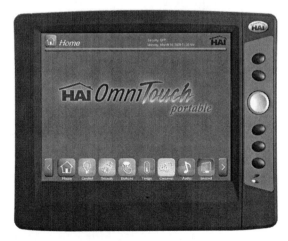

HAI OmniTouch 10p,
www.homeauto.com
Device for controlling your home automation.

automation professionals, and as you can probably guess, they are expensive. But the flip side is that you can automate as much or as little of your home as you wish.

CLUE

Web Search
Search for the following terms:
home automation installation [your city]

Here are some popular categories for home automation:

✓ **Lighting.** Put lights on timers or activate via motion sensors.

✓ **Heating and cooling.** Manage the temperature in your home with an electronic thermostat. More complex systems can program different temperatures for different rooms at different times of the day.

✓ **Safety.** Automate and integrate home safety features such as intrusion detection or smoke and carbon monoxide alarms.

✓ **Entertainment.** Integrate all of your audio and video equipment so that you can control it from one central location.

The really nice home automation systems include slick easy-to-use controllers. For example, the HAI products (see www.homeauto.com) can be controlled by a really snazzy touch-screen with a lovely interface. The fancier the system, the more it's going to cost. A top-of-the line system can run in the tens-of-thousands of dollars. However, you could also choose to upgrade only your thermostats or lighting for a few hundred.

Door Handles

It's the small things that can make a big difference.

Small round door handles can be impossible to grasp and turn for people with severe arthritis. That's why they make door knob grippers—special devices that fit over the door handle to allow necessary grip and leverage to turn the knob.

You can buy a Door Knob Gripper from The Wright Stuff (shown here) for a scant $5.95. It seems a small price to pay to be able to move freely in your own home.

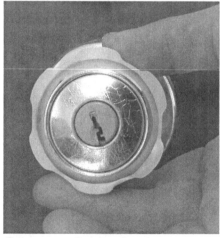

Grippers make opening doors easy

Smart Toilet

It was bound to happen. Senior Technology has found its way to the toilet.

Let me be the first to introduce you to the Neorest 600, a breakthrough in toilet technology from the company Toto.

This toilet includes a number of really fantastic features:

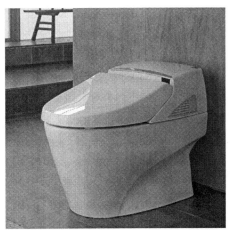

High-tech toilets are here at last. The Neorest 600.

✓ Sensors detect when you are near and automatically open and close the toilet lid

✓ Automatic flushing

✓ Wireless remote to control: water for hands free cleaning, water temperature, warm air dryer, air purifier, and self-cleaning feature

This toilet is pricey (several thousands of dollars), but if you have extra money lying around and want to treat yourself to a luxurious bathroom experience, check it out.

Toto also produces the Washlet product —a seat that attaches to your existing toilet and uses warm water to clean up post-toileting. The Washlet 300 allows you to program the temperature of the seat, the cleansing water temperature, and the force of the water. Although it may seem a little extreme at first blush, this product (and others like it) can offer assistance to those seniors who need a little extra help in the bathroom.

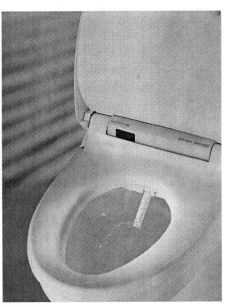

The Toto Washlet seat fits onto your existing toilet.

The Toto Washlet product line features a number of products at different price points—from a few hundred dollars to near a thousand.

Hearing Aids

What?

I said, "HEARING AIDS!"

You would have heard me if you had been wearing the latest and greatest hearing aids.

These things really work well, and with electronics getting smaller and smaller each year they are virtually invisible. In addition, these gadgets take advantage of digital signal processing to improve the user's experience. Here are a few advantages of digital signal processing:

✓ Controls the "gain" to limit sudden loud sounds (like a car horn). Previously, the sound would have just been amplified and hurt your ear.

✓ Cancels out background noise (such as the din of a 747 flying above) so you can hear more important things like speech.

✓ Enhances speech by boosting the frequencies of the human voice.

✓ Directional microphones can improve your experience, mimicking the natural collection of sound in a healthy ear.

Hearing aids are, however, expensive and are not (for some mind-boggling reason) covered by most health insurances. But there really is no question about it—if you need hearing aids and can afford them, you must get them. Don't be discouraged by some misperceived stigma against hearing aids. For one thing, you can barely see these tiny devices. But more importantly, no social stigma is worth surrendering one of your senses.

Healthy hearing helps us maintain relationships and experience the world around us. Don't miss out.

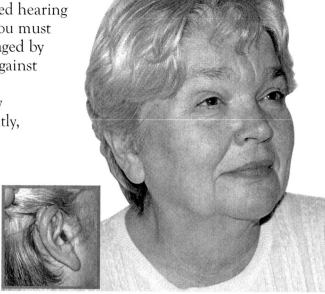

Practically invisible modern hearing aids.

Robots!

What could simplify your chores more than someone (or something) else doing them for you? Nothing! And that's why God made robots.

I'm not talking about those sci-fi humanoid machines that will someday take over the planet. I'm talking about task-specific smart devices that perform everyday chores like vacuuming your carpet or mowing your lawn.

Here are a couple of robots so helpful that everyone—not just seniors—should have them.

iRobot's Roomba

iRobot was the first company that put robotic floor cleaners on the map. "Why do I need a robot to clean my floor?" you ask.

Because it can. And it does a darned good job of it.

Now before you go picturing Robby the Robot running around with a broom and dustpan, I should set some expectations. Roomba is a small circular machine that stands only a few inches tall. Actually, it doesn't "stand" at all—it rolls.

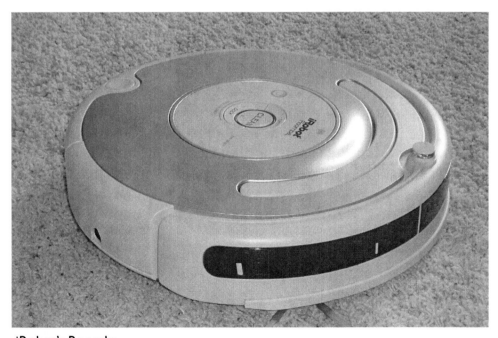

iRobot's Roomba

This little cylinder powers itself up at a preprogrammed time and then zooms around the room in a semi-random pattern. When it hits a wall it follows it. When it hits a chair leg, it goes around it. At the end of the process, after it has covered the entire floor, the Roomba returns to its station to recharge.

This is really nifty. But before you get too excited there are a few things to note.

✓ You'll need to empty the Roomba periodically.

✓ A Roomba is really only rated to clean a moderately sized floor—think two to three rooms max. If you have a lot more floor space, you might need two Roombas.

✓ These machines are quite hearty, but they will need maintenance every few years.

The best part is the price. Prices range from $150 to $600. The more expensive models have a few bells and whistles (such as scheduling) and typically clean more on a single charge. But the entry-level machines still do a great job and save you the trouble of vacuuming.

I love these things.

TIP-OFF

If you try and enjoy the Roomba, you should also consider getting iRobot's floor washing robot—the Scooba.

Wheelchair-Mounted Robotic Arm

Researchers are developing solution after solution for people with severe mobility issues. One solution is the wheelchair-mounted robotic arm. This would allow the driver to grasp items on the ground or above the chair. A few companies—for example Phybotics located in New Jersey—have already created these types of wheelchairs, but they are not yet available to the mass market.

Going one step further, researchers at the University of South Florida have integrated the wheelchair-mounted robotic arm with a Brain Control Interface (BCI). This allows the user to control the arm just by thinking about it. Again, this is far from production, but the possibilities for increased mobility and independence are staggering.

If you think you'll want one of these in, say, 10 years from now, you better start saving your money now. They will not be cheap.

Active Exoskeleton

The Institute for Human and Machine Cognition (IMHC) in Pensacola, FL is currently developing an assistive walking device—a powered exoskeleton that adds extra energy to your motion. Imagine sprinting up stairs again.

Or performing 20 minutes of deep knee bends (not sure why you would want to do so many knee bends, but with the Active Exoskeleton you could).

In the prototype, the exoskeleton straps comfortably to your legs and is powered by a tethered power source.

Sounds great, right? You bet! Watch out for this type of product to really revolutionize senior mobility.

Check out their website for more information and to see some videos of their exoskeletons in operation.

www.ihmc.us

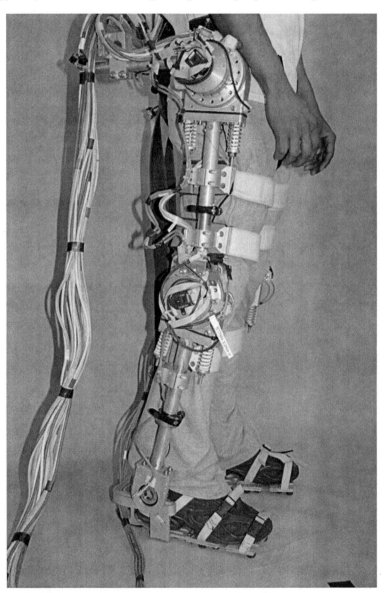

The IMHC Active Exoskeletorn prototype adds strength to help the user walk up stairs.

Robotic Lawnmower

Similar to the Roomba (the squat device that cleans your floor) the robotic lawnmower is a squat device that—surprise, surprise!—mows your lawn. These battery powered robots feature self-charging stations and scheduling capabilities and are smart enough to cover an entire lawn (up to about ¾ acre) when unleashed.

These things cost several thousands of dollars—easily twice as expensive as regular self-propelled lawn mowers. But they are cheaper than paying someone to mow your lawn, with a payback period of between 1 and 2 years.

Setup is somewhat involved, requiring you to lay (or bury) a perimeter wire so that the robot knows where to mow. And maintenance can also be tricky—lots of moving parts to break. But overall, consumers seem happy with these products.

If interested, check out some reviews on the following robots:

- Zucchetti-Lawnbott ($4500)
- Friendly Robotics-Robomower RL 1000 ($2500)

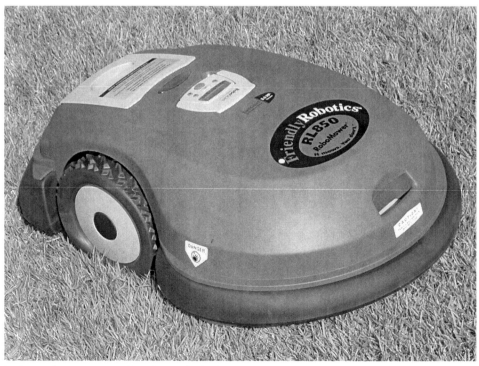

Robotic lawn mower (model RL850) from Friendly Robitics..

Home Monitoring

You don't need home monitoring. You'll be fine—living a thousand years without ever facing a medical emergency or a fall.

Actually, I lied.

The real statistics for home-emergencies for seniors are a bit more grim.

Roughly one-third of seniors fall each year. Some of these falls only bruise your body and ego—others can lead to serious problems. The key to getting through a really nasty fall or other home health emergency is quick response. The quicker you can get help, the better you chances are for a quick recovery.

Even if you are one of the 66% of seniors who don't fall this year, that doesn't mean that your friends and family aren't going to worry about you.

And that's why we have home monitoring technologies—to alert friends and family if and when you have a home emergency. Home monitoring adds another layer of home safety for you and helps your family feel more comfortable with you living independently.

Monitoring (and Preventing) Falls

According to the Technology Research for Independent Living (TRIL) Center, over 30% of people 65 and older fall each year, with 12% of these people falling twice. Falls lead to broken bones. Broken bones can lead to hospital stays. Hospital stays can lead to infection. Infection can lead to longer hospital stays or worse.

It's really best not to fall.

But if you do fall, there are some nifty technologies that will send for help.

Preventing Falls

We all trip. And there ain't no technology that's going to fix that—except maybe a proximity alert sensor mounted to our feet that screams, "watch out, stupid!" before you kick the bed frame.

But falls are also caused by balance, strength and cognition issues associated with aging. These types of falls we can try to prevent. Here are a few nifty technologies currently in the works to help prevent falls.

iShoe

Researchers are developing an electronic device worn in the shoe that analyzes your balance to detect chronic balance problems early—before you fall. Your doctor will be able to recommend balance treatment based on the iShoe tracking results.

It's easy to imagine this product taking one more step (pardon the pun) forward to actually alert you before you fall to give you a chance to recover balance.

This product, being developed by a team at MIT, is still in the prototype stage. It could be available as early as 2010 and estimates place the cost at around $100.

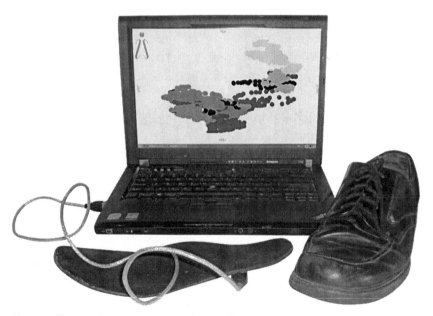

iShoe will provide computer analysis of your balance.

Vibrating Shoes

A number of companies and research centers (MIT among them) are also researching the effects of a vibrating insole. They contend that the vibration stimulates nerves in your foot, which improves balance and reaction time.

Look for products marketing this technology by 2011.

Human Airbag

OK, so this isn't really a preventative technology, and it sounds kind of goofy, but it's real.

A Japanese company has developed a human airbag to cushion your impact if you do fall. Sensors in the airbag vest detect when you are falling and inflate within 0.1 seconds, providing a soft airy impact.

Note that the airbag only protects you if you fall backwards. Also note that the current list price is around $1000.

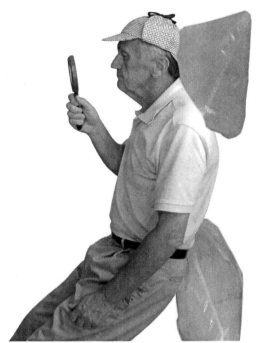

Even a Senior Sleuth can fall. The human airbag could literally save your butt.

Alerting for Falls

Unlike fall prevention technologies which are still in the development stage, fall alert technologies are already here. They come in two basic flavors:

✓ **Manual (push-button) alarms.** Seniors wear devices on their person; these devices feature large easy-to-push buttons that send an alert when activated.

✓ **Automatic alerts.** The latest generation of fall-alert technologies do not rely on anyone pushing a button; rather they detect a fall through sensors either on the person or somewhere in their home (such as their carpet).

Note that these devices are all currently limited to home use within range of a centralized receiver. It's not hard to imagine, however, these devices integrating with cell phones in the near future to provide fully mobile alerting.

Manual Alerts

Push button alerts are sold with a subscription to a monitoring service. If you fall (and I hope you don't), you simply push the button on your emergency call button. A live voice then inquires as to your status through a separate speaker system.

A few points are worth mentioning.

✓ Most manual alert systems are designed for use in the home. You—or rather your call button—needs to be within a certain range of the speaker system, which in turn needs to be connected to your phone line.

✓ This technology is subscription based. You'll pay a little more than a dollar a day for the service. This differs slightly depending on the company or product you select.

There are dozens of push-button alarms available. Here are just a few examples.

Product/Company	Description	Cost/month
Lifeline Medical Alert	Wearable pendant or Timex watch integrates with a call box or special phone. The call button is waterproof and so can be worn in the shower. `philips.lifelinesystems.com`	$35
LifeResponseUSA	Similar features to the Lifeline product, but this wearable pendant is arguably less stylish than the Lifeline. This company offers free equipment, free shipping and free support. `www.liferesponseusa.com`	$25–$35
LifeStation	Similar features. Call button can be worn as necklace, watch or on the belt.	$30 (with options to add additional buttons or call services)

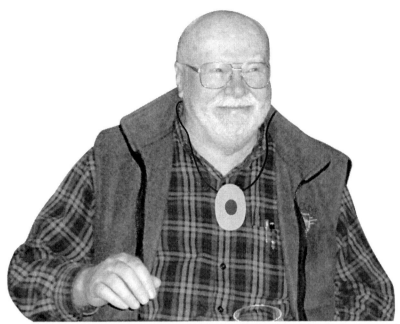

Some push-button pendants are worn around the neck for easy access in case of emergency.

Automatic Alerts

There are several available technologies that can detect when someone falls and then send an alert to a monitoring service or individual. These automatic alerting technologies come in the following forms.

Sensors on Body

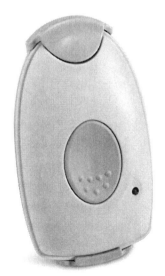

Sensors worn on the body can detect the signature motion of falling. When a fall is detected in the home, the device automatically sends a message to both the call center and optionally to family or friends through text messaging or a phone call.

Here are a few companies featuring automatic fall alerting. Both provide the equipment for free—you just need to pay the monthly subscription fee.

BrickHouse Alert fall detector device worn on your person automatically detects falls and calls for help.

Automatic Alert Product	Description
HaloMonitoring myHalo	A sensor is mounted to a comfortable strap that you wear around your chest. In addition to detecting falls, the device also monitors other vitals such as heart rate and body temperature.
	This product requires broadband to work effectively, but still works during a power outage.
	Can automatically send a text message, update a web page, or call contacts in addition to the call center.
	www.halomonitoring.com
BrickHouse Alert	Clip to your belt or clothing or wear it as a pendant around your neck.
	In addition to the fall alert, this system comes with an intruder alarm and includes live reminder calls (e.g., for taking medication).
	Routes all calls through the call center. The call center representative can then connect you to other people in your contact list.
	www.brickhousealert.com

Floor Sensors

Companies are currently developing special flooring that can detect when you fall. A team at the University of Missouri is developing one such product called the "Smart Carpet." It uses a thin sheet of sensors between your carpet and carpet pad to track and analyze your traffic pattern and detect falls. This carpet could then be hooked up to an automatic alert service to quickly dispatch help if you need it.

Look for this product to be in stores by 2011.

Monitoring for Activity

Two more signs of senior trouble—actually, they're signs for any-aged trouble—are inactivity or irregular activity. If you don't get out of bed for two days in a row, that's probably a bad sign. More frequent trips to the bathroom could also indicate something has gone wrong. Recognizing inactivity or significant changes in behavior can tip off doctors and caregivers to a problem before it escalates into an emergency.

Fortunately, a few home-based systems do just this. Motion sensors are mounted strategically throughout the home and networked through a computer. After some configuration and time for learning your routine, the integrated computer notes any major changes in your activity. It then sends alerts when it detects a problem.

Let's investigate two well-advertised options for home monitoring. Both of these products use strategically placed motion sensors to monitor and track movement through the house. This can include, for example, a motion sensor near your bed to ensure you get out of bed or a sensor by your pill box to make sure you've taken your medication on time. When your daily pattern deviates, alerts are automatically sent to care providers

Product	Description
QuietCare	Company Information: Located in New York City, they boast the first commercially available monitoring system. Differentiating Features: ✓ Bathroom fall detection. If you are inactive in the bathroom for too long, the system assumes you have fallen. ✓ Does not require a computer in the senior's home. All information is routed through a special receiving box, connected to the Internet through a standard phone line. ✓ Web-based alerts and reports Website: www.quietcaresystems.com

Product	Description
IngeniumCare	Company Information: Located in Denver, CO. This company will launch its signature product in Summer 2009. Differentiating Features: ✓ Fall detection by wearable pendant. ✓ Reminders and medical verification ✓ Includes vital sign monitoring ✓ Can integrate with other home automations such as heating, lighting, and security systems Website: www.ingeniumcare.com

Monitoring for Cognition

Your brain is another essential tool for successful independent living. This should not surprise you. Our brains are important—especially for Senior Sleuths!

Don't believe me? Use that brain of yours to research important brain functions.

Unfortunately our brains are subject to effects of aging. They slow down. They get more forgetful. And they can get sick. Cognitive deterioration can lead to a host of other physical and psychological issues, such as accident proneness, missing medication, malnutrition, and depression.

Detecting cognitive issues early can lead to successful treatments, which ultimately results in a healthier, happier you. This is why a number of research organizations and companies are working on products that provide an unobtrusive way of monitoring our cognitive health.

For example, scientists from the Oregon Health and Science University have shown that existing computer card games can be tweaked to monitor someone's cognitive health. The way they play the game—how fast they finish as well as how they finish—provides key insights into how their brains are working. This study was done in conjunction with a private company called Spry Learning, Inc. who may turn the results into an unobtrusive cognitive evaluation tool.

It's easy to imagine this technology infiltrating other software applications and popular websites. You perform a task—play a game or fill out your tax forms—and the software analyzes your brain health. The most obvious place for early integration will be in brain-training software.

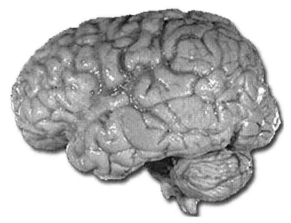

The brain is an important—though somewhat slimy—part of every senior body.

Unfortunately, as of this printing there were not yet any proven products commercially available. But it's only a matter of time before there are explicit cognitive monitoring software applications that quietly monitor your brain health as you go about your normal business.

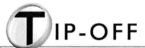 **TIP-OFF**

The Technology Research for Independent Living (TRIL) has a number of projects investigating cognitive functions. One such proposed project, which they call Dear Diary, is a system that can detect cognitive problems through speech analyses. Imagine speaking into a computer and the computer diagnosing any issue instantly.

Truth be told, it's a little scary. I wouldn't want to get bad news from a computer. If they ever perfect this technology I hope they soften any bad news by giving the computer a smooth soothing voice.

Visit www.trilcentre.org to learn more.

Visual Monitoring

Visual monitoring is probably the most obvious form of home monitoring. Cameras are cheap and they can be easily integrated with your computer. You can set up networked cameras in your kitchen, bedroom, bathroom, and any other room in the house. Your friends and family can keep a close eye on you for a teeny tiny investment with little setup. Yep. Cheap and easy.

It's also mildly creepy.

Do you really want your kids and grandkids logging onto their computer just in time to see you sit down on the toilet? Or changing your clothes? Or making a sandwich?

I don't, but that's just me. For some people this is an acceptable alternative to losing your independence. They will allow the occasional prying eyes if that will help their kids feel more comfortable with them living alone.

Here's a quick list of pros and cons to visual monitoring.

Pros—I look good in the buff:

✛ No recurring fees. You buy the small cameras, install them around the house, hook them up to your computer and you're done. No subscription fees.

✛ Guaranteed to spot an emergency. If you fall, someone will see it. If you accidentally stick yourself in the refrigerator, someone will see it.

Cons—God made clothes for an obvious reason:

▬ Installation is difficult. You need to mount cameras and then wire them to the computer. You can outsource this to a technician, but it'll cost you.

▬ Someone has to be watching the video feed in order to spot a problem. There is no automatic alert sent when something goes wrong. A fall, for example.

▬ Does not work in a power outage.

▬ Feels more like an invasion of privacy than any of the other home monitoring technologies. (This may not be a problem for you if you are a life-long exhibitionist.)

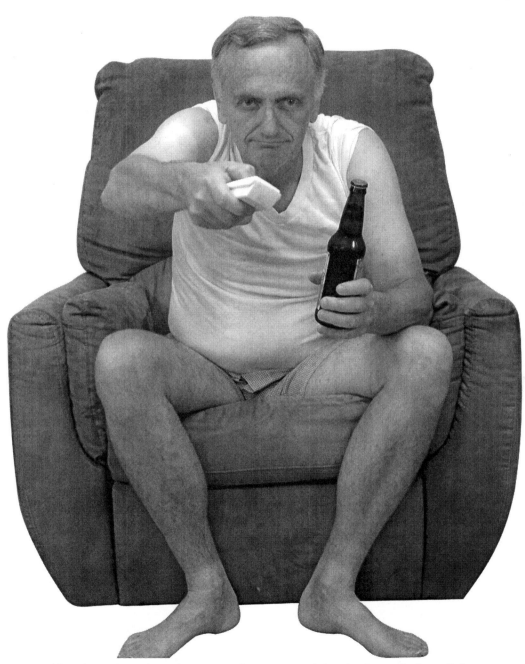

Visual monitors let others see what you are doing (and wearing) at all times.

Communication

Nothing beats sitting around a campfire with your grandkids chatting about sports, politics, and the latest TV craze. This is communication at its best—when you can see expressions, share a roasted marshmallow and just relax and talk. Ahhh...

Unfortunately, you can't have a campfire every night. And even if you could, you certainly couldn't expect your kids and grandkids to be available every night, or to be as enthusiastic as you are about maintaining a deep relationship seasoned by the smell of campfire. People have their own interests, their own free-time activities. That's what makes them interesting.

Campfires are great. So are family dinners, reunions, and trips to the Grand Canyon. But these won't satisfy all of your basic communication needs. Fortunately, there are new technologies for staying in touch and developing relationships with friends and family.

New modes of communication are predicated on the old modes. We still connect through speaking, writing and looking; but technology has added a new flavor and immediacy to these "conversations."

The following technologies offer a very real opportunity to connect with more loved ones more often—even if they live on the other side of the planet. These are not substitutions for face time. They are supplements. We can't be together all the time, but we can stay much closer by using the new communication technologies.

In this chapter you will investigate:

➢ Phones

- ✦ Cell Phones
- ✦ Phones over the Internet
- ✦ Senior Phones
- ✦ Smart Phones
- ✦ Texting

➢ Online Communication

- ✦ Email
- ✦ Instant Messaging
- ✦ Social Network Websites
- ✦ Twitter
- ✦ Video Chat

Background Check

It's hard to believe that 150 years ago the only way to get a message across the country was by giving a letter to a guy on a horse. This is how our great-grandparents communicated with distant relatives. A lot has changed since then.

1856
Western Union Telegraph Company begins operations.

1876
Alexander Graham Bell invents telephone and sends the message "Mr. Watson, come here. I want to see you." It is the first message sent over his new telephone system.

1878
First Commercial telephone switchboard.

1887
The USA has 150,00 phones lines; UK 26,00 and France 9,000.

1889
The first Pay Phone is installed in Hartford, Connecticut. Each call costs 5 cents.

1892
The first direct dial phone goes into service in La Porte, Indiana. (Fifth Information Revolution)

1915
First coast-to-coast telephone conversation in the United States.

1950
Bell Labs and Western Electric create the first telephone answering machine.

1956
AT&T lays the first Transatlantic telephone cable (Scotland to Newfoundland)

1969
ARPANET, precursor to the Internet, goes online at UCLA, Stanford, and the University of Utah.

1972
First basic email program created for ARPANET.

1977
Fiber-optic telephone cables are installed.

1991
World Wide Web begins. First web camera used at Cambridge University—it was pointed at the coffee pot in the computer science department.

1995
America Online, CompuServe, and Prodigy begin offering dial-up internet service.

1997
Camera phone is invented.

2002
Friendster founded—first popular social networking site.

2003
MySpace is created (later sold in 2005 for $580 million)

2004
Facebook founded.

2005
Skype offers free video conferencing across the internet using webcams.

2006
Twitter product created—gained massive popularity in 2007.

2007
Apple releases the iPhone.

Phones

Yes, I realize that you already know what a phone is. You call someone, you have a conversation, you hang up, you pay your bill. And that's all there is to it. Right? Not by a long shot.

Modern phones are complex electrical devices, which often incorporate a number of non-phone features like cameras and Internet browsers. Phones also have different ways of making calls—some home phones use the phone line, some use an Internet connection, some use wireless cell towers, and some even use satellites.

Let's take a look at the different flavors of modern telephone.

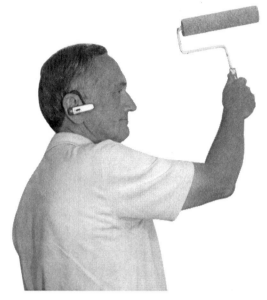

Wireless bluetooth device connects to your phone, sits in ear and frees your hands for other "fun" activities.

Cell Phones

Portable. Wireless. Fantastic.

The modern cell phone began in the late 1970's as a large wireless car phone that could send and receive signals to nearby cell towers. As electronic components shrank and batteries became more powerful through the following decades, so did the cell phone. By the early 1990's cell phones were small and light enough to carry around on your person. Since then phones have gotten smaller, lighter, and are jam packed with additional features.

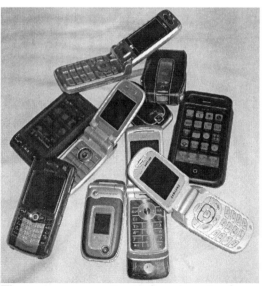

There are many options when shopping for a phone.

How to Buy a Cell Phone

You can't just buy a cell phone and expect it to magically work. In fact, you can't just buy a cell phone—you need to also buy a phone plan. The phone plan determines which cell phone service provider carries your calls, how many minutes of talk time you get and which geographical regions you can call.

And then you need to consider the phone features and quality. Does the phone have everything you need? Maybe you need a "smart phone" for your Senior Sleuthing activities—to take pictures of secret documents and to upload them to your sleuthing web page. Does the phone meet your physical needs? Maybe you need bigger keys because your hands are a little shaky, or maybe you need an external volume setting for easier listening.

When shopping for a cell phone, consider the following:

✓ **Features**—Do you want Internet access, music players or other non-phone features in your phone?

✓ **Usability**—How is the call quality? Is there an easy-to-access volume control? Are the buttons big enough to push only one at a time?

✓ **Cost**—How much does the phone cost? How much does the plan cost?

Reception—Will your cell phone get a signal at your

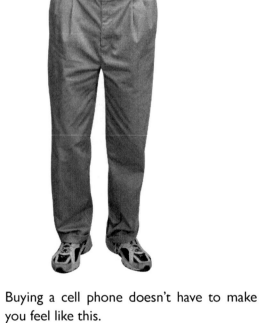

Buying a cell phone doesn't have to make you feel like this.

home and other places you frequently visit?

You need to answer each of these questions before committing to a cell phone contract. Oh yeah... they make you sign a contract for one or more years. But don't let this discourage you from getting a cell phone. They are extremely convenient and relatively affordable. Once you get one, you won't mind being under contract. In fact, you'll renew without a second thought when the time comes.

Cell Phone Plan Options and Considerations

Here are some items common to many cell phone plans.

✓ **Number of Free Minutes.** Many plans offer free night and weekend talk time.

✓ **Number of "Anytime" minutes.** This is how many minutes you are allotted during non-free times.

✓ **Family Plan.** Share minutes with one or more family members. This is cheaper than buying two individual plans.

✓ **Rollover minutes.** Unused minutes can be used in subsequent months. If you only used 300 of your 400 allotted minutes for the month, you'll have 500 minutes (400 + 100) at the start of the next month. Rollover minutes typically expire after a year.

✓ **Free long distance.** Any good plan will offer free long distance calls. They'll subtract minutes, but they won't charge you long distance rates for the call.

✓ **Texting options.** Sending text messages uses a slightly different communication protocol and so providers charge you for it. You can sign up for a certain number of text messages per month, unlimited text messaging, or can pay per text message sent.

✓ **Mobile to mobile (also called "friends and family") feature.** Pick a certain number of people that you can call without using minutes. This is a great option if you have a handful of people that you call most often.

✓ **Data plan.** If you buy an Internet-ready phone (like the Apple iPhone) and intend on accessing the Internet, then you'll need a data plan. This allows you to surf the web and send emails from your phone.

Each plan will have its benefits laid out in a nice bulleted list.

Where to Buy

You can buy cell phones in physical stores (electronics stores or stores run by the service providers) or online stores. Purchasing in person is usually easier as the sales guy can walk you through all of the plan options. Purchasing online will almost always get you a better deal.

If you're buying in a bricks-and-mortar store, then just check your yellow pages for a store near you. If you're buying online, then there are hundreds of sites where you can buy a cell phone and plan.

Here are just a few options:

Web Page	Comments
www.amazon.com	Features customer reviews for most phones and plans.
www.letstalk.com	Specialty cell phone shopping site. There are many of these sites on the Web. Before purchasing from one of these sites, make sure it is legitimate. You can look for a company review on www.bizrate.com.
www.apple.com/iphone	If you want to buy an iPhone, you need to purchase it through the Apple or AT&T websites. See store.apple.com/iphone for more information on this exciting product.

Where to Read Reviews

There are a number of websites that provide in-depth reviews of cell phones. These are extremely helpful when shopping for one of your own. You'll see how others rate items like reception, usability, and design. I usually skim the review for any red flags for my personal needs. If, for example, the phone does not include an external volume control, then I'll move to the next model. If, however, there are complaints about the display brightness, I might let that slide. I'm more sensitive to hearing issues than sight issues.

Here are a few sites that provide cell phone reviews and rankings.

Web Page	Comments
`www.consumerreports.org`	Although you must pay to see the rankings on this site, it might be worth the fee. Consumer Reports tests a lot of products back to back and so can effectively rate based on relatively scientific criteria.
`www.cnet.com`	CNET provides Editor's reviews for many products. If they have a review on your cell phone, then you're in luck. This will tell you all the good, bad and ugly of the phone.
`www.amazon.com`	Use Amazon to see what other actual users think about the product. These are not trained reviewers, so you'll get a wide range of review quality.
`www.google.com`	If all else fails, try a Web search. Search for "[cell phone model] review" and watch as a dozen reviews pop up on the search results. Take note of who is reviewing the product. Be suspicious of any product reviews coming from the product manufacturer's site.

Home Phones Using Your Internet Connection

There is a cheaper way to make calls from your home—assuming you have a high-speed Internet connection. You can now make phone calls over the Internet. This technology is called Voice Over Internet Protocol, Voice Over IP, or VoIP.

Voice Over IP allows you to make unlimited calls to any other phone in the world for a reasonable flat rate. If you have family and friends all over the world and plan to talk to them regularly, this might be a useful technology for you.

There are, however, a few things to consider before full adoption. Here's a quick list of pros and cons to VoIP technology.

VoIP Pros:

✦ **Cost.** Inexpensive monthly rate that includes most (if not all) call charges. Depending on your service, there may be a small premium charge for long distance or international calls, but these charges are still less than half of standard phone-based calling plans.

✦ **Portability.** You can plug your special IP phone into any high speed Internet connection and retain the same phone number. Heading down to Florida for the winter? Take your IP phone, plug it in, and your friends and family can reach you at the same telephone number.

TIP-OFF

VoIP phones will not work during power outages, so if you expect to need help when the lights go out, this is probably not the right technology for you.

VoIP Cons:

— **Useless during a power outage.** If your power is knocked out by a big storm, you're on your own. Normal phones are powered through the phone line and don't rely on power in your home. VoIP phones must be powered to work. Note that if you have an emergency call system that relies on a phone connection, you can't use VoIP.

— **Special phone.** You may have to purchase a special VoIP phone. These are generally more expensive than normal phones, but not prohibitively so. More VoIP phones are coming onto the market all the time, so this problem is becoming less of an issue.

There are a number of VoIP companies and you can easily find them with a simple web search for "VoIP." Providers include Vonage, Phone Power, Lingo, and ViaTalk.

Phones Designed for Seniors

With every sector of manufacturing looking to bust into the senior market, it should come as no surprise that there are already phones designed specifically for seniors. This typically translates into better audio options, simplified menus (for cell phones), bigger buttons, and an easy-to-read display.

The following table lists a few manufactures and products to consider if you're interested in a senior-friendly phone.

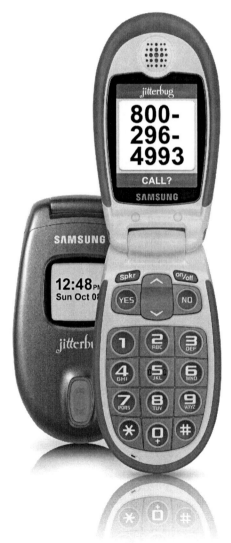

The Jitterbug cell phone is designed for seniors.

Phone	Comments
Jitterbug	Simplified cell phone with flexible service plans—pay for minutes now or pay as you go. They don't have contracts, which is great. The downside of this is that you have to pay the full price of the phone, which runs around $150. This phone features: ✓ Large keys modeled after classic telephone ✓ 24 hour operator who can help you place calls Note that your minutes don't roll-over. They expire after 90 days. Also, this phone has limited international access (i.e. calling from a foreign country could be a problem). `www.jitterbug.com`
ClarityLife C900	Simplified cell phone with a number of senior-friendly features. This is an "unlocked" phone, meaning that it will work with most carriers after you insert that carrier's electronic card into it. The cost for this phone is around $185. This phone features: ✓ Emergency call button on back of phone—calls up to five programmable contacts. Note that it does NOT call 911. ✓ Can be amplified to twice as loud as a regular cell phone ✓ Text messaging available ✓ Includes flashlight. Clarity also manufactures dozens of other amplified phones for the home. Check out their website at `www.clarityproducts.com` to see their full offering.

Super High-Tech Phones (Smart Phones)

There are a number of phones marketed at high-tech junkies and business powers. These "smart phones" feature advanced touch screen displays, integrated cameras, music and video players, web searching, maps and GPS, and multiple downloadable software programs.

There is no reason why seniors can't enjoy all of these over-the-top techno features. You take pictures. You watch videos. You surf the Web. You want to know your GPS coordinates.

Two of the most popular smart phones are the Apple iPhone and the Blackberry. Both phones feature the full gamut of "smart" features.

The iPhone is recognized by most people to have the slickest user interface. This phone featured one of the first (certainly the most popular) touch screen phone interfaces. For example, you can zoom in on a picture by pinching the screen. How neat is that?

The Blackberry is still reigning champ among business users. Blackberries offer a nice interface for synchronizing data with Microsoft Windows office software—specifically Microsoft Exchange email program.

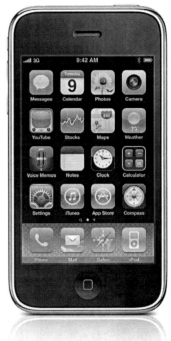

Apple iPhone features a slick touch-screen interface.

Texting: A Primer

"Texting" refers to sending short text messages from one cell phone to another. Because these text messages were originally constrained to 160 characters, text messaging is still sometimes referred to as SMS (Short Message Service).

People who grew up with this technology on their phones are ridiculously fast at typing messages on the phone's keypad. Remember that for most phones you don't have a full QWERTY keyboard to bang out the messages—you need to navigate the number pad, which has three or four letters per key. If you've got a grandkid that's a good texter, ask him to show you how he sends a message. It'll knock your socks off.

In order to compensate for the awkward keys and character constraint, a new texting language has emerged. There are thousands of texting abbreviations and there are new ones popping up every minute. If someone sends you a text with an abbreviation that you don't understand, just Google it.

Here are a few popular text-isms that might pop up on your display.

Text Abbreviation	Meaning
?	I have a question.
411	Information.
404	I don't know.
AYDY	Are you done yet?
B2W	Back to work.
CU	See you.
DUR	Do you remember?
EZ	Easy.
F2F	Face to face.
GTG	Got to go.
HAGN	Have a good night.
IMO	In my opinion.
JK	Just kidding
LOL	Laugh out loud.
NRN	No response necessary.
OOTD	One of these days.
PMFI	Pardon me for interrupting.
QQ	Quick question.
SUL	See you later.
TBH	To be honest.
VN	Very nice.
WBS	Write back soon.
ZZZZ	Sleeping or bored.

If you want to send a text to a friend and happen to be sitting by a computer, you can save a little time by using a free web utility to send the message for you. You can simply type your message on your normal keyboard and send it. Much faster (at least for me). One such website is www.textforfree.net.

Communicating Online

The Internet has opened doors to new and exciting avenues of communication. Written online communication is faster and easier than sending a letter via the post office (now called "snail mail"). And online audio and video communication gives you a way to chat and look at each other without requiring expensive video equipment.

Online communication is just plain cool—and it's free with an Internet connection.

Online communication now comes in three flavors:

✓ Email

✓ Instant Messaging (IM) and Online Chat

✓ Social Networking Websites

Email

Email (short for electronic mail) provides near-instant communication between two computers. Each email user has an email "address" where they can receive correspondences. For example, if you send an email to the address seniorsleuth@gmail.com, it will go to one of our Senior Sleuth editors.

Your email address is included in each email you send, so it's easy for recipients to quickly reply to your mail.

Email is sent over the Internet using an email software program or free email service hosted on a Web page. Two of the most popular free email services are Google Mail (Gmail) and Yahoo Mail. For each of these services, you need to create an account and select a username (which translates into your email address) before sending mail. It takes about two minutes to create an account.

Your high-speed Internet provider will also include a few free email accounts with your subscription. These are fine, but if you ever decide to change your

Internet provider (for example, you move out of state), then you can't take your email address with you. For this reason, it's probably a good idea to use one of the free web-based email services.

With Gmail and Yahoo you can access your email from any computer with Internet access. Just go to the email web page, log onto your account, and read and send mail.

As with their search pages, Google and Yahoo mail pages also include advertisements. These are relatively unobtrusive and you quickly learn to ignore them.

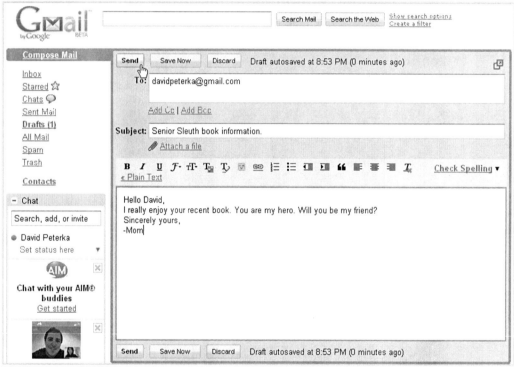

Gmail is a popular (and free) email tool.

The New Tone

Emails are less formal than classic written correspondences. An email to a friend could be as short as one sentence or one word. And you'll be surprised at how many people include misspellings and relaxed (some might argue incorrect) styles such as sending a message with all lower-caps.

If, however, you are sending an email to a prospective employer, then you should make every effort to present yourself in a formal and professional manner.

Email is fast and so quality is often sacrificed for speed. This is not a judgment—just letting you know what to expect.

Email Attachments

You can attach just about any computer file to your emails. This allows you to share documents, photos, and other data with friends and families. You do, however, need to be cautious when opening attachments from other people—especially from unknown sources. You could accidentally open a computer virus that wreaks havoc on your machine. Don't worry about this too much. Most email services scan your attachments to ensure they are virus free before letting you open them.

Spam!

Spam is another word for unsolicited junk email. These are usually some sort of advertisements for products or services. Left unchecked, you might receive several hundred spam emails every day. Fortunately, most email services include a spam filter—technology for automatically deleting or sequestering the junk emails.

When you receive a spam email, you can (and should) mark it as a spam message—usually by clicking a **Spam** button on your email page. This will help your email system filter out other similar spam messages in the future.

TIP-OFF

Advertisements beside your email

Some free email services (like Yahoo and Google mail) display advertisements on your screen. They do this by scanning your email and placing advertisements related to the content of your message. This raises some alarms for privacy experts, who think that your correspondences should be seen by you and only you. Others don't mind a computer reading their mail.

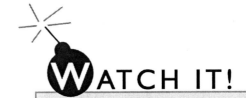

WATCH IT!

Whatever you do, NEVER click links or open attachments contained in spam emails. These will most certainly be annoying (or lewd) and could potentially be dangerous to your computer. Trust me on this one.

Modus Operandi

How to send an email from Google Mail (Gmail):

Sending emails from Google Mail (or Gmail) is easy. Here's how to do it.

1. Open a Web browser (like Internet Explorer).
2. Enter `mail.google.com` in the Web address field and click **Enter**. The Gmail sign in page opens.

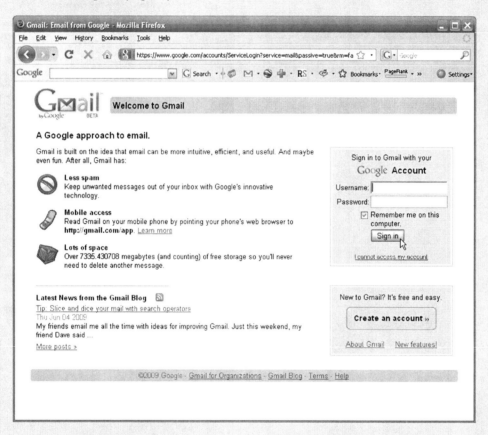

3. If you DO NOT have an account, click the **Create an account** button to create a Username and Password.
4. If you DO have an account, enter your `Username` and `Password`.

5. Click **Sign in**.

   The main Gmail page opens.

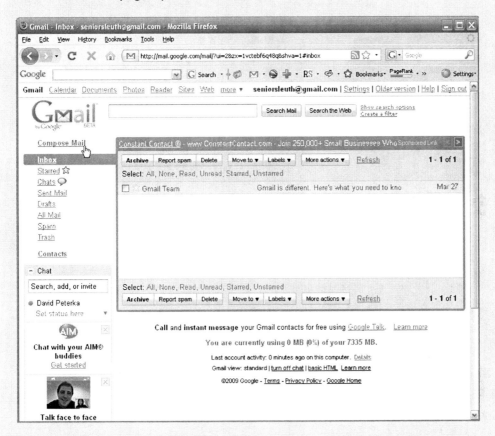

6. Click **Compose Mail**.

   A blank email page opens.

7. In the To: field, enter the email address for the person you want to email.

   Email addresses have the format [name]@[provider].com. For example, seniorsleuth@gmail.com.

8. In the Subject field, enter an optional quick description of your note.

9. In the large white text area, type the body of your message.

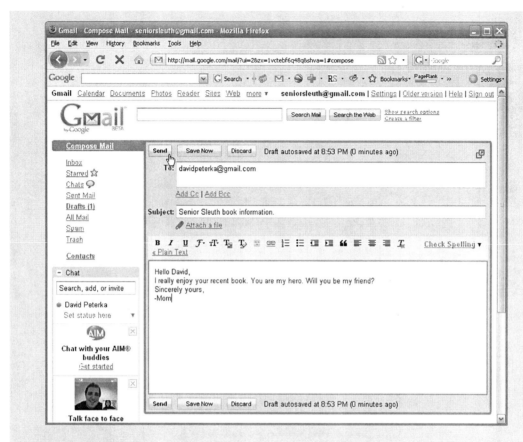

10. Click **Send**.

And off the email goes. The recipient (the person specified in the To: field) will receive the message in a few seconds.

Instant Messaging (IM) and Online Chat

Instant messaging (IM), also called online chat, is a text-based technology that allows you to have a back-and-forth conversation in real-time through a specialized messaging software. Using the IM software, you can see which of your contacts are online and available to chat. From there, you simply send a message to the person you want to chat with. They respond with their message. And this process repeats until you either get bored with each other or are called away.

Check out an example (on the next page) of an online chat between myself and a Senior Sleuth editor using Google chat, Google's free IM program.

Instant Messaging Networks

Most email service providers also include an Instant Message service. Three big names that provide IM access are Windows Live Messenger (Microsoft), Google Chat, and Yahoo Messenger. This allows you to have one account from which to send both emails and IM's. There is, however, a drawback to using the email provider's IM—you can only chat with other people using the IM service through that provider. For example, Google chat users can only instant message with other Google chat users.

This might not be a problem for you—especially if all of your contacts use the same email program (for example Google Mail). If, however, you have friends using all different types

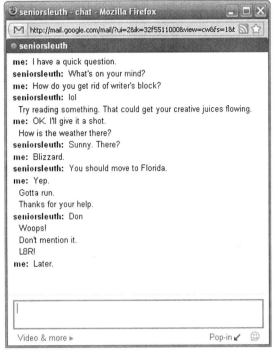

Quick chat with the Senior Sleuth using Google Mail's built-in (and free) chat software.

of IM software, then you might consider using one of the following IM services that allow you to chat with people on different networks.

Digsby	www.digsby.com
Pidgin	www.pidgin.im
Meebo	www.meebo.com

Each of these IM programs is free, making money (presumably) through their on-screen advertisements. All received positive user and expert reviews.

Note that Meebo is a browser-based program, meaning that you can access your IM account from any computer with a modern web browser on it (which is just about every computer).

IM Abbreviations

IM chat abbreviations are similar to cell phone text messaging abbreviations. In fact, many abbreviations are the same. For example, you might see someone type **lol** (laugh out loud) in both phone text messages and computer IMs.

Here's a short list of common IM abbreviations. Note that these abbreviations often provide shorthand for either phrases you might say in active conversation or status updates.

Text Abbreviation	Meaning
ATM	At the moment.
BRB	Be right back.
CUL	See you later.
GG	Got to go.
IMHO	In my humble opinion.
JK	Just kidding.
L8R	Later.
NP	No problem.
SYS	See you soon.
TTYL	Talk to you later.
YT?	You there?

Social Networking Sites

Social networking sites are websites where people who share similar interests can form, maintain or nurture relationships—both personal and professional. Social network users create their own pages containing personal information and can grant others permission access to those pages. Similarly, friends (or people with similar interests) post their information and grant other people access to their spaces.

What types of information do people share on their pages?

People typically list their interests (such as favorite films, books, and sports) and include a few personal historical tidbits (such as high school or college) on their page. This allows other social network users to find people with similar interests and background. For example, you might search for and befriend someone in your graduating high school class. Or maybe you want to join a Humphrey Bogart fan club.

The number of groups (or small social networks) that have popped up on these sites is staggering. If you can think of a group, there probably is one already. If not, then you can easily create it and invite others to join.

The two most popular social networking sites are Facebook and MySpace. There are other social networking sites out there such as Friendster, but most new users are flocking to the two sites discussed below. And if the point is to socialize, why not go where everyone else is going?

MySpace (www.myspace.com)

MySpace has been around longer and therefore has more U.S. members than its main rival Facebook. MySpace was the first mega-networking site where the general public could post information about themselves and search for other people with similar interests.

MySpace features a flexible interface where you can customize your page (also called your "space") to create a unique look and feel. It helps to know HTML (the programming language for creating web pages), but even if you don't, you can still make the page unique.

As with almost all online services, you need to create an account before using MySpace. This takes between 5 and 10 minutes. Then you can spend countless hours, days and months customizing your page and looking through others'.

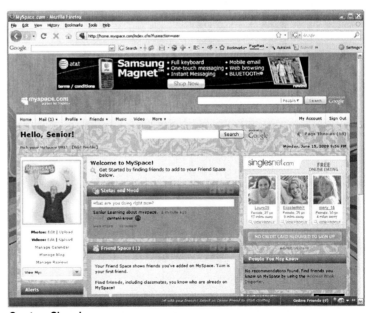

Senior Sleuth myspace page.

Facebook (www.facebook.com)

Facebook is the new kid on the block, but as of 2008 it had surpassed MySpace for the largest number of global users. And if it continues along its current trend, it will surpass MySpace for U.S. users sometime in 2010.

Facebook has similar features to MySpace. You can post pictures, music, videos. You can search for people based on geography and interest. So why are more people using Facebook?

Word on the street is that it's easier to use and looks better. It also offers a couple of other nice features that appear to be attracting users:

✓ You can post your status on your "wall," where your friends can see it and add comments of their own.

✓ You can track your friends' updates through a news feed. When they update their status, you see it on your feed.

✓ You can easily "tag" someone in a photo and that picture will be shared with all of the tag-ee's friends.

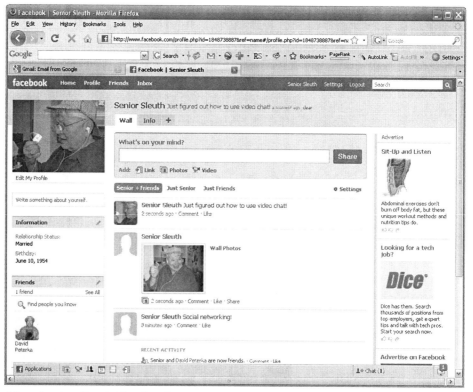

New Senior Sleuth Facebook page.

Which One? Facebook or MySpace

Which one is better for the senior?

It depends on which one your friends and family are using. If they are on MySpace, then you should definitely have an account there. If they are on Facebook, get a Facebook account. But here's the real magic—you can have an account on both! Remember that this is a way to see what your friends are doing and to give them some insight into your life. Both services are free, so why not try both?

But if you had to choose only one social network, I would probably pick Facebook. The interface is less busy and more interactive. I like seeing when my friends make updates, so the news feed is a must have for me.

Modus Operandi

How to post your status on your Facebook Wall:

Facebook allows you to post your status—a short statement of how you're feeling, what you're doing, or what you are thinking about. Your status will appear on your friends' Facebook home pages.

1. Open a Web browser (like Internet Explorer).

2. Enter `www.facebook.com` in the Web address field and click **Enter**.

   The Facebook login page opens.

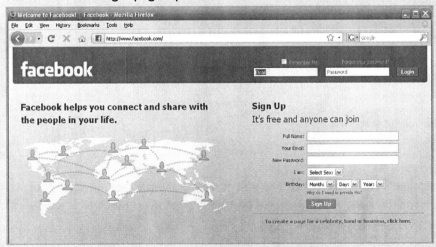

3. If you do NOT have an account, enter your information in the Sign Up fields and click **Sign Up** to create your Facebook account.

4. If you DO have an account, enter your `Email` and `Password` at the top of the page and click **Login**.

Your Facebook Home page opens.

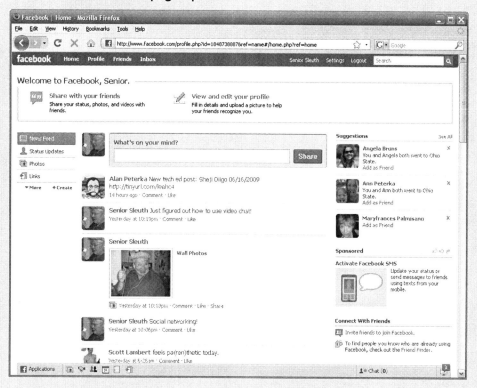

5. In the `What's on your mind?` field, enter a brief status.

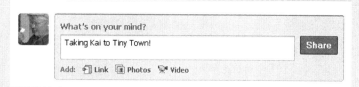

6. Click **Share**.

Your new status appears just below where you entered it. You can update your status as frequently as you want. Facebook aficionados might post an update every hour. More casual users post updates a few times a week or less.

Twitter (www.twitter.com)

Twitter is a service that can send short messages (140 characters or less) from your phone or computer to anyone who subscribes to receive your messages. The messages are called "tweets."

To use Twitter you post your tweets to your Twitter page. Twitter does the rest—sending it out to anyone who "follows" your page.

Q: But why?

A: Because it's neat.

Q: What can you say in 140 characters?

A: Plenty—if you are crafty.

Much like text messages or IM and Social Network statuses, Twitter gives you the power to let people know what you are doing right now. Tell friends and family what you're reading, how long you've been waiting for your plane, your thoughts on a surprising news story. These won't be deep commentaries on life and culture, but they will give others a window into your life.

Twitter can be easily integrated with social networking sites like Facebook. You can automatically post your tweets for your non-Twitter social network to see.

Twitter sounds goofy at first, but it can be fun. Give it a try. It's free.

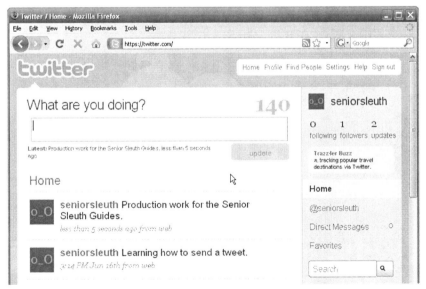

The Twitter web page where you can post your tweets.

MODUS OPERANDI

How to send a Tweet:

Tweets are often sent using the texting (SMS) features on cell phones. The cell phone user sends a text message to their Twitter account and that "Tweet" gets distributed to anyone who has subscribed to follow your postings.

You can also send a tweet from the Twitter website. Here's how to do it.

1. Open a Web browser (like Internet Explorer).

2. Enter `www.twitter.com` in the Web address field and click **Enter** on your keyboard. The Twitter sign in page opens.

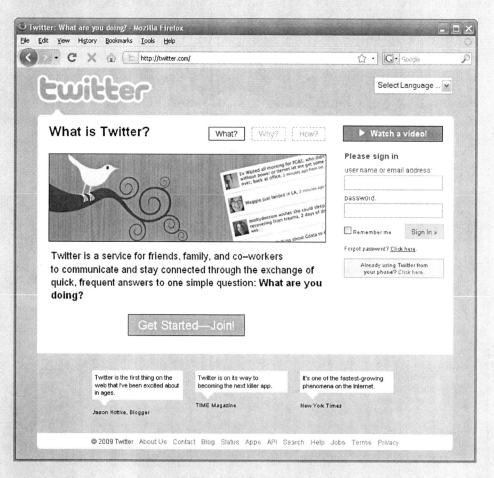

3. If you do NOT have an account click **Get Started—Join!** to create a Twitter account. It only takes a few minutes to sign up.

4. If you DO have an account, enter your username or email address and Password at the top of the page and click **Sign In**.

Your Twitter Home page opens.

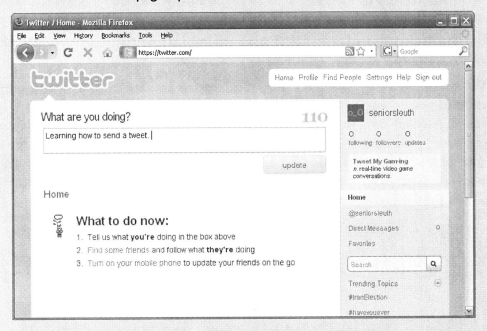

5. In the What are you doing? section, enter your 140 character or less tweet.

6. Click **Update.**

Your new tweet appears just below where you entered it. You can tweet as frequently as you want. Twitter aficionados might tweet every hour. More casual users tweet a few times a week or less.

Anyone who "follows" your tweets will receive your tweet within a few seconds.

TIP: The above process is for tweeting through the Twitter website. You can also send tweets from a cell phone using the phone's "texting" feature.

Online Video Conferencing

What if you just aren't satisfied with talking on your high-tech cell phone or sending IMs and tweets to friends and family? What if you actually want to look at your grandkids to see how they are growing?

Well, you should go visit them. No substitute for that. See Chapter 7 Travel and Transport for senior travel technologies.

But for those of us who do NOT have unending travel funds, there is another option: video conferencing.

Video conferencing (or video chat) sends video and audio of you sitting in front of your computer to another computer over the Internet (and vice versa). A small camera mounted on your computer or built into your laptop captures video and an external or internal computer microphone captures your voice. Video and audio are then routed through special software, which is installed on both computers. The end result—you can see and hear the

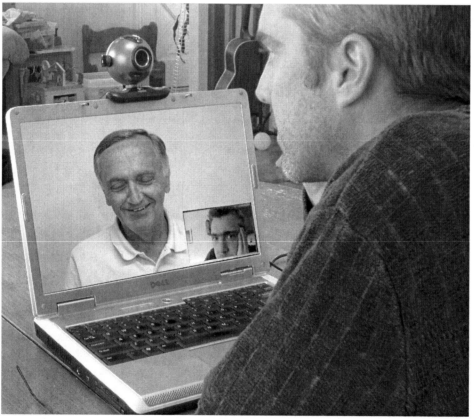

Connect with family and friends using a free video chat program over the Internet.

person you are talking to.

The set up is a little tricky. You'll need the following items in addition to your computer and high-speed Internet connection:

✓ Webcam (or web video camera) – prices range from $20 to $200

✓ Microphone – $5 to $50

✓ Online chat software and account – free through a few companies, most notably MSN and Skype. Visit their websites for more information.

Technology	Description	Cost
Webcam	Small video camera that can be easily mounted to your computer monitor or set on your desk. These plug into a common port in you computer and usually require you to install accompanying software "drivers." Some computers have a webcam built in to the computer. You can buy these from any electronics store, though you'll find a better deal if you purchase online. Don't forget to read reviews before buying!	$20 - $200
Microphone	External microphone that plugs into either the computer's microphone input or into a USB port. I recommend buying a microphone built specifically for your PC. They will come with a nice desktop stand for easy positioning. Note that some laptops include built-in mics. If yours does, you don't need to buy one.	$5 to $50
Online chat software and account.	A few companies provide free video chat capabilities. Two notable companies are Microsoft (through Windows Live Messenger) and Skype. Both are easy to install and use. Once your camera and microphone are installed, simply open Windows Live Messenger or Skype and initiate a video call. The first time you do this you'll be led through a short process to make sure your camera and microphone are working.	Free

Installation and setup for video chat
is all relatively easy, though you do
need to get everything right before
it will work. Most webcams include
excellent instructions for not only
setting up their device, but also
setting up a video conference. Some
companies charge for their own
video chat service. Although the
connection quality is probably better
for the pay services, the free ones are
good enough. And they're free. All

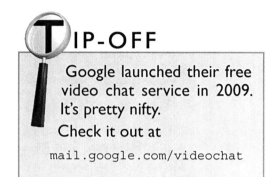

TIP-OFF

Google launched their free
video chat service in 2009.
It's pretty nifty.
Check it out at
`mail.google.com/videochat`

they'll cost is a little installation effort—a little sweat power. In my opinion,
it's worth the expended elbow grease.

Your Privacy on the Internet

When you use the Internet, other people and companies might be able to see
some of your data. Companies often use this data to tailor product offerings
to you. "Nice" people might want to casually see how you are doing or where
you live; "naughty" people might try to use your data for nefarious purposes
such as identity theft.

It's all about balance—finding the right level of information sharing to allow
family and friends to see what you are up to, while discouraging the evildoers
from destroying your credit.

When thinking about Internet privacy, we typically consider the following
two categories:

✓ Privacy with Online Vendors

✓ Privacy on Social Networking Sites

Privacy with Online Vendors

When you use the Internet, some of your personal information is seen (or
collected) by Websites and online vendors. For example, when you search for
a book on Amazon.com, they store information related to your visit—namely,
which books you looked at—in either a cookie (a file on your computer) or in
their database (if you have logged onto their site).

Most online vendors have a lengthy privacy statement, which usually includes the following points:

✓ They will use your personal information (such as buying habits) to analyze sales trends and to, as they put it, "better deliver the goods you want to see." For example, if Amazon knows which types of books you bought on your last visit, then they can use your personal information to display similar books on your next visit.

✓ They will NOT sell your personal information to a third party.

✓ They will NOT give your financial information (credit card number and billing address) to anyone. They usually take great care in protecting this information and making sure all of their financial transactions are "secure."

Should you be concerned?

Probably not. In fact, you may find that this data collection is really convenient. For example, you love to travel and book a flight to some exotic destination every month using an online travel reservation website. (It's nice to be you.) Because you have created an account on Orbitz, you no longer need to enter your personal information (for example, payment information) when you book your tickets. Orbitz has already collected it and stored it in its

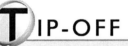

TIP-OFF

You can turn OFF Internet cookies, thus limiting how much information you automatically share with online vendors.

For example, using the Firefox web browser, select **Tools > Options** from the menu and click the **Privacy** button on options screen.

You can then uncheck the box for "Accept cookies from sites" to restrict vendors from tracking your information on subsequent visits.

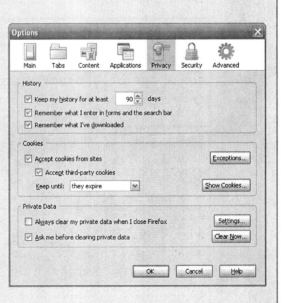

secure database. This saves time and gets you on that plane to Hawaii with a little less hassle.

But not all online vendors are so careful with your private data. Most of the big stores will act responsibly, but if you decide to purchase something through a lesser known site, make sure to read their Privacy Statement, which is usually linked from their Home page. If you don't see it and can't find it, then that's probably a good indication to shop somewhere else.

Privacy and Social Network Sites

Privacy concerns have a slightly different twist on social networking sites. Rather than worrying about companies automatically storing information about your online activities, social network privacy is concerned more with the level of public access to your personal page or space.

For example, when you create a Facebook account, your page is (by default) private—meaning that only you and invited friends can see your information, pictures, status updates. On the flip side, when you sign up for Twitter, your page is (by default) public—meaning that anyone with computer access can see your page.

All of the prominent social networking sites allow you to change your privacy settings. The following table summarizes the default privacy settings for the top three social networking sites.

Social Network	Default Privacy	How To Change
Facebook	Private (only Friends can see your info)	From the top of the page select **Settings > Privacy Settings**. On the resulting page, click on **Profile** to set who can see your information.
MySpace	Public (everyone can see your info)	From your MySpace home, click the **My Account** link. On the resulting page, click **Privacy** to restrict who can see your information.
Twitter	Public	From your Twitter page, click the **Settings** link. At the bottom of the resulting page, click the box for **Protect my tweets**. This will allow only approved people access to your tweets.

Travel and Transport

Any Senior Sleuth worth his weight will be up to date on current transportation technologies. How else will you tail your suspect as he hops a train to Miami? Or skip town when you are framed for an untoward crime? Or book a cruise online for your wedding anniversary?

A huge number of seniors travel. In fact, travel ranks at the top of leisure activities for people over 50. Seniors travel more frequently and stay at their destinations longer than younger generations. It's no wonder there are so many delightful senior travel technologies.

So which technologies make Senior Travel a better experience? Computers, the Internet, and slick new manufacturing techniques have given us a host of gadgets that make getting from here to there faster, safer, and cheaper.

Background Check

Travel and transportation technologies have been evolving ever since the first prehistoric human slipped his foot into a leather bag to protect his foot from cold and rocks. Since then we've developed shoes with integrated electronics, planes, trains, automobiles, and complex computer-based travel booking and tracking systems.

Look at the next page for a high-level timeline of some major milestones in travel and transportation technology.

Planes, Trains, and Cruises

Seniors make up 80% of all luxury travelers in the United States. Prior to the Internet, you had to either limit travel to familiar destinations or book your trips through a seasoned travel agent. But now you can research and book a trip to virtually any corner of the globe from your own kitchen table.

Let's investigate two applications of how the Internet has broadened our travel horizons.

Researching Destinations Online

As a Senior Sleuth you understand the old adage, "knowledge is power." This is especially true when planning a vacation. If you could somehow research hotels at your destination or compare different cruise ships, then you could all but ensure a great vacation (not counting any negative effects of weather, illness, lousy company, or a bad golf game).

Luckily for all of us, there are a number of online resources for researching travel destinations before you go. Here are just a few.

TripAdvisor (www.TripAdvisor.com)

TripAdvisor provides travel recommendations for accommodations, vacations, and travel packages. This is all well and good, but the real power of TripAdvisor is its enormous selection of user reviews.

Interested in going to the beautiful island of Maui, but don't know where to stay? Your first stop should be TripAdvisor. Click the Hotels tab at the top of the web page and then search for Maui. Dozens of results are returned. Click on any of the results to read the reviews of people who have actually stayed

	Shoe Tech	Car Tech	Plane Tech
8000 BC	8000 BC Earliest shoe in archeological data.		
	1300 AD Straps and laces added to shoe.		
		1769 First self-propelled (steam) vehicle created by Nicolas Cugnot.	
			1793 Jean-Pierre Blanchard made the first balloon ascent in the United States.
			1848 Henson and Stringfellow built a steam-powered model aircraft, which flew 40 meters before crashing—marking the first heavier-than-air powered flight.
	1899 Patent for rubber heel on shoe.	1885 Gottlieb Daimler invented the prototype of the modern gas engine.	1877 First flight of a steam-driven model helicopter (Enrico Forlanini).
		1908 First model T created.	1903 The Wright Brothers made first controlled, powered heavier-than-air flight at Kitty Hawk, North Carolina.
		1911 GM introduced the electric starter.	
		1913 Ford introduced conveyer belt assembly.	
	1917 First sneaker (soft-topped shoe).	1915 Ford Motor Company built one-millionth model T.	
			1919 First non-stop transatlantic flight.
		1939 Buick added electric turn signals to cars.	1939 First jet aircraft created for the German Air Force.
			1947 Chuck Yeager broke the sound barrier.
		1951 Chrysler introduced power steering.	
		1953 Air conditioning included in cars.	
		1955 Seatbelts first required in Illinois.	
		1959 Three-point seatbelts invented.	
	1970 Odor-eaters invented.		1970 Boeing created the 707, the first wide-bodied plane.
	1980 Nike began manufacturing shoes in China.		
		1982 First Japanese company (Honda) began making cars in the U.S. (in Ohio).	
		1997 Toyota created first hybrid (gas-electric) Prius.	
		2006 Tesla produced completely electric car.	2007 Airbus A380, the largest passenger airliner in the world, made its first commercial flight.
	2008 Nike integrated with iPod to track runs while providing music.	2008 U.S. auto manufacturers faced serious financial problems.	
2010		2009 President Obama declared new efficiency standards for autos.	

there. For most popular destinations, you'll see well over a hundred user reviews.

This approach shares the power of Amazon user product reviews, but it also shares the same limitation—namely that anyone can write the review, including the property management. So you need to take the reviews with a grain of salt. There is, however, a certain safety in numbers. If two-hundred reviews are negative and five are glowing, then you should steer clear.

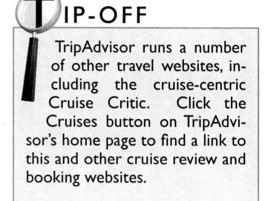

TIP-OFF

TripAdvisor runs a number of other travel websites, including the cruise-centric Cruise Critic. Click the Cruises button on TripAdvisor's home page to find a link to this and other cruise review and booking websites.

TripAdvisor is currently the most popular travel review site, and therefore has the most customer-driven data. This is a must-stop website for any trip planning.

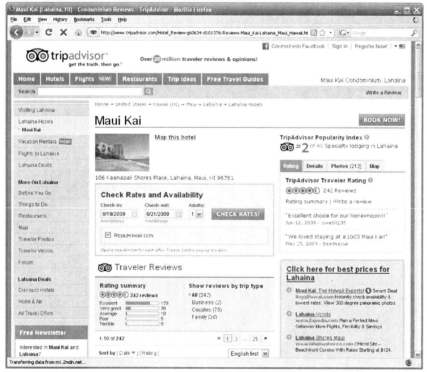

Maui Kai hotel receives hundreds of "Excellent" reviews on TripAdvisor.

Reviews on Travel Booking Sites

There are several websites where you can book flights, hotels, cars and cruises. We'll discuss these in more detail in a later section. Although I strongly recommend using review sites like TripAdvisor to research any accommodations before booking, you can also read select reviews on the actual booking site before purchasing your tickets or reservations.

For example, when you search for Hotels in Maui using a popular travel reservation website like Orbitz (`www.orbitz.com`), each hotel listing includes a link for user reviews. This is a great feature and you should read the reviews. You will notice, however, that there are far fewer reviews on these sites compared to TripAdvisor.

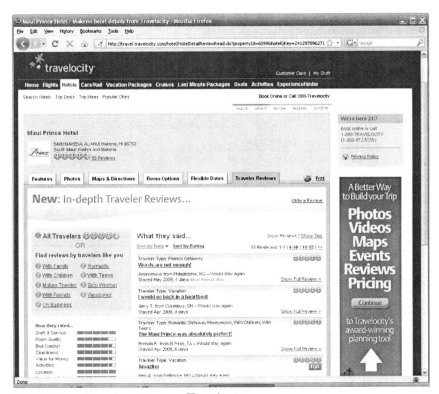

Maui Prince Hotel reviews on Travelocity.

U.S. Department of State (http://travel.state.gov/)

Safety should be a factor in any international trip. The U.S. State Department provides an up-to-date listing of foreign countries with dangerous travel conditions. This can include countries with increased violence or hostility toward Americans, areas with escalated risks of exposure to disease, or countries with damaged infrastructure.

You should always check the State Department's list of travel warnings and travel alerts before leaving the country. Links to these travel advisories are located at the top of the state department's web page.

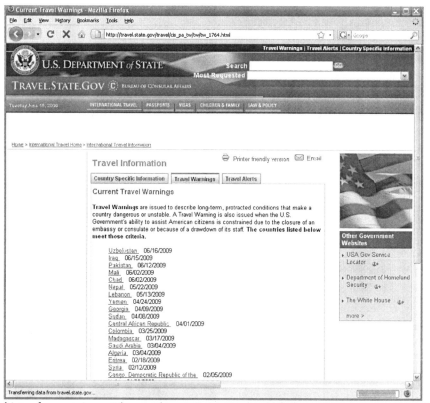

List of countries with travel warnings on the U.S. State Department's website. From this page, you can click the country name to see the full report.

Travel Reservation Websites

Now that you've researched your destinations and have planned the perfect trip, you just need to buy your tickets and reserve your accommodations.

No problem. Just head over to your favorite online travel reservation websites, search for a flight, hotel, or car, and book it!

The travel sites return a number of results matching your search parameters. For example, you search for a flight from Denver to Orlando and the search yields 100 possible flights—prices ranging from $200 for a flight with a layover in Atlanta, to $725 for a direct flight. Simply skim through the results for the one that best fits your need and budget.

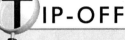

TIP-OFF

Note that many airlines do not post all of their inexpensive fares more than a few months in advance. If you're not finding any great deals—even with the flexible date option—wait a few weeks and try again.

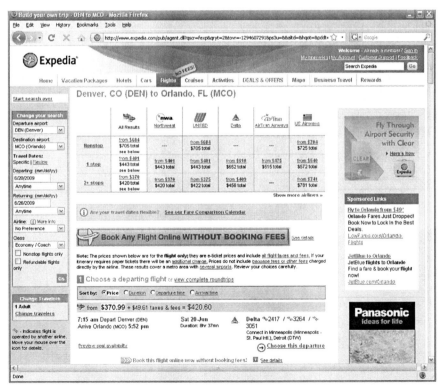

Expedia flight search results for flights from Denver to Orlando.

Popular Travel Reservation Websites

Here's a quick list of the top 5 travel reservation sites (according to several online surveys). Use any of these sites to quickly find great deals on travel.

Site Features	Expedia	Orbitz	Travelocity	Priceline	Hotwire
Flights	X	X	X	X	X
Cars	X	X	X	X	X
Hotels	X	X	X	X	X
Cruises	X	X	X	X	X
Trains		X	X		
Flexible Dates	X	X	X		
Direct flights	X	X	X		

TIP-OFF

One more travel reservation website worth mentioning is Kayak. com. This website searches for travel deals and itineraries posted on other reservation sites, as well as the airlines' websites. Kayak also does a nice job of presenting your travel options in a grid for- mat so you can instantly see the benefits of flexibility—for example, shifting your travel dates by one day might cut your ticket price in half. Kayak.com is my favorite flight booking site.

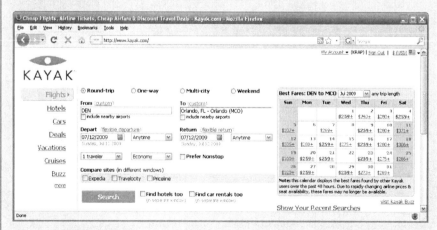

Tips, Tricks and Gotchas

Here are a few tricks for booking trips online. I've also included a couple of annoying "gotchas" that you are sure to encounter if you frequent these sites.

Flexible Dates

If your travel dates are flexible, you can probably save a great deal of money on your trip. For example, you might find that mid-week flights are cheaper than weekend flights. You might also find that travel to, say, Florida is cheaper in April rather than in March.

Most of the online reservation websites listed above provide an option to search for fares over a large range of dates. For example, you could search for all flights between today and June 30th and then sort the results based on price to find the best deal. Searching for specific dates will almost always return higher ticket prices.

I recommend searching for a large range and then selecting your trip dates based on the best fares.

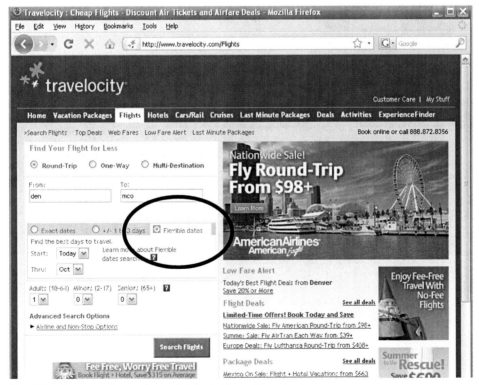

Flexible dates option selected (circled) on Travelocity.

Nearby Airports

Many online reservation websites allow you to search for flights into and out of airports in proximity to your selected airports. For example, you want to fly from Denver to Cleveland. You select the "search nearby airports" option and then you are shown fares from not only the Denver and Cleveland airports, but also Colorado Springs (near Denver) and Detroit (near Cleveland). If the fares to and from the nearby airports are much less expensive, you can then decide whether it's worth it for you to travel in and out of the alternate airports.

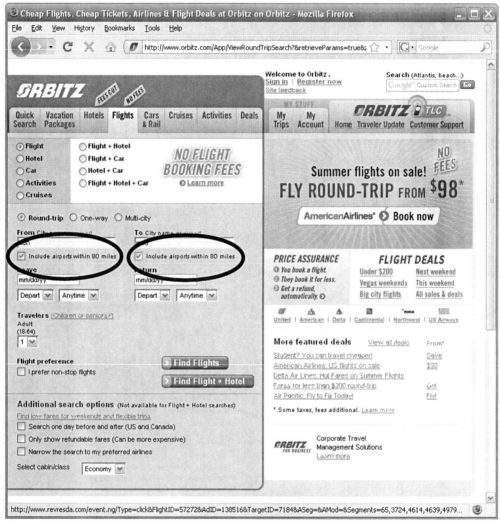

Include nearby airports option selected (circled) on Orbitz.

THE JIG IS UP!

Fare No Longer Available!?!

This is the most annoying feature of the online reservation websites. You search for a flight between cities and find a great ticket price. You click on the link to buy the ticket and then the website says something like, "We're sorry. The fare you selected is no longer available."

Worse—you might not even get the courtesy of that message; rather, you'll spend half an hour clicking on a bunch of travel dates, only to find out that all seats are sold out. (See picture below. The X's denote that the seats are sold out.)

The website operators claim that this is the airline's fault—some nonsense about the airline not keeping their schedules current. I don't buy it. I hold the website responsible. If they can check the actual fare AFTER I click the link, why can't they validate availability BEFORE I click the link? It feels like a bait and switch every time. And it's a waste of my time.

Whenever this happens on a search site, I simply take my business elsewhere.

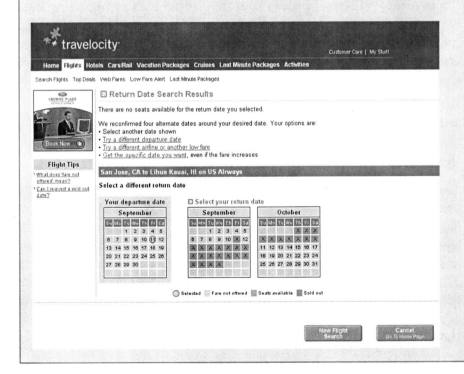

Feet Technology

Walking is the oldest mode of transportation. (OK—I suppose it's the second oldest, after crawling.) You'd think that as we get older, we would just get better and better at it. Unfortunately, our joints can wear down and our balance can falter.

And when walking gets more difficult, our first instinct is to do less of it. This is the wrong approach. As the saying goes, you have to "use it or lose it." Walking is great exercise—good for body and soul. You should do it as much as possible.

For those of us with more serious mobility issues, there are some technologies that can help. The following sections present some great advancements to help encourage exercise and enable greater mobility.

High-Tech Shoes

Humans have come a long way since the days when we slipped a leather bag over our feet and called it footwear. Now shoes are more fashionable, comfortable, therapeutic, and sometimes even electronic!

We've already discussed shoes that help avoid falls by analyzing balance issues and vibrating the insoles to improve balance. See Chapter 5 for more information on these shoe technologies. Rather than duplicating content and wasting precious investigative page space, let's consider another high-tech shoe option for seniors: the Nike+ system.

Although marketed to runners, the Nike+ system is a perfect Senior Technology.

What is it?

The Nike+ shoe integrates with an iPod (music player) to measure how far and fast you walk or run. After your run, you upload the data to your computer where previous walks or runs are logged. This provides you with a record of your exercise and allows you to analyze your performance, calorie consumption and overall cardio fitness.

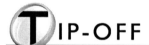

TIP-OFF

Nike and Apple are already working on the next generation of this technology, which (according to their patent) could include actual GPS tracking and sensors in the shoe to notify you when you should replace them.

How does it work?

The current model includes a small pocket inside the shoe where you place a tiny pebble-sized accelerometer. The accelerometer sends data wirelessly to your iPod (or special wristwatch), which logs your movement. This data is then uploaded to Nike's website, where you can see lovely graphs and charts of your performance.

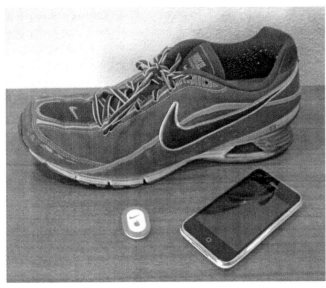

Shoe sensor button, iPod and shoe are all you need to track your runs or walks with the Nike+ iPod solution.

Why would I want one of these?

This is the fancy version of carrying a pedometer. It tells you how far and fast you travel and highlights trends in your fitness. For me, these shoes provide extra motivation when exercising. Now that I know how fast and far I can walk, I like to match or beat my previous distance or time. It also gave me a good excuse to go out and buy an iPod music player.

The shoes and sensors aren't particularly expensive (as far as shoes and electronics go), but you do need to own an iPod device (Nano, Touch or iPhone). Here's the cost breakdown using the iPod Nano.

Running shoe:	less than $100
Nike+ iPod Sport Kit:	$30
iPod Nano:	$200

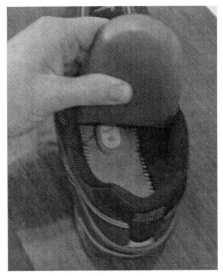

Shoe sensor button, sits unnoticed underneath the Nike's insole. You won't even feel it—I promise.

The Cane

Should your sight fail in your senior years, you could take advantage of the latest interesting technological twist on the classic cane—sonar! Much like a bat locating insects in the dark, this cane notifies the operator of obstacles by bouncing sound off of them. The cane registers different shapes at different distances with a different sound/pitch sent to the operator.

See the following website for more information: www.batforblind.co.nz.

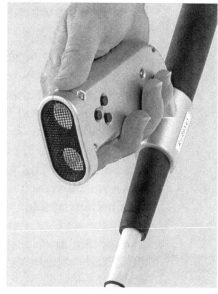

Signals sent and received from the cane's grip.

Walkers

Today's walkers are better than walkers manufactured even 10 years ago. The reason for this is simple: better materials. Manufacturing companies can now utilize the latest breakthroughs of material science and build their products stronger and lighter than ever before. And for walkers, lighter is better.

But there are even more interesting walker advances on the horizon. Here's one example of a high-tech walker poised to hit the market.

I-walker

A group of researchers at the Technical University of Catalonia have designed a walker that can respond to its environment and communicate with the user. For example, the walker could learn the mobility

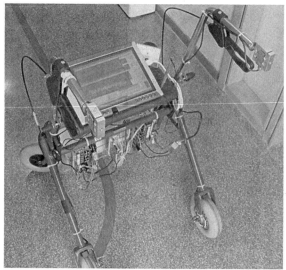

The iWalker (still in development).

constraints of the user and warn the user if he is nearing his distance limit. The walker could also respond to voice commands such as, "take me to the kitchen." The walker would then lead you to the kitchen.

These are still in the design phase. Look for this type of smart walker to be available by 2011.

A better hip!

The human body is not immune to wear and tear. A lifetime of use can wreak havoc on any body part—especially the ones that support our full body weight. I present to you Exhibit A: the human hip.

With life spans increasing, there is a good chance that you're going to outlive your hip. So what do you do then? Simple. You get a new one.

Until recently, hip replacement surgery was an in-patient operation which required several days in the hospital followed by several months of intense rehabilitation at home. But now a new anterior replacement procedure can be performed with as little as a one-day hospital stay and full recovery in as little as 2 weeks.

The newest operation goes through the patient's front side through a natural space between muscles. Because the surgeon doesn't cut through or detach muscle, the healing time from the operation is greatly accelerated. Additionally, patient movement is not restricted following surgery. This is better than the conventional surgery where patients are warned against such basic movements as crossing their legs, which could lead to a dislocation.

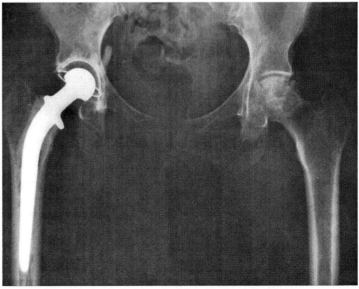

New hip can increase mobility and improve life.

There are fewer doctors trained in this surgical method, so you may have to travel to get this operation done. If you want less pain and faster recovery (and the doctors tell you that you are eligible for this type of operation), then I strongly recommend it.

Navigation—Handheld GPS

With Global Positioning System (GPS) devices, you will never get lost again. You can now use a handheld device to show your current position overlaid onto a city or topographical map. This comes in handy when walking around an unfamiliar city or when hiking a new nature trail. Most of these devices also display points of interest, restaurants, and stores. So if you're wandering around in London and want to grab a bite to eat, check out your GPS device to find all eateries within two blocks of your current location.

These GPS devices will not only show your current location, but they are also loaded with a number of cool features, such as providing precise directions between two points or measuring the distance and rate of your afternoon hike.

Most GPS devices come with some built-in maps, but you'll want to make sure you have complete coverage for the city or park you plan on exploring. Knowing your latitude and longitude doesn't help as much as knowing a cross street for city navigation.

As with all technology, there is a huge price range for these devices. Higher price usually indicates more features—not necessarily better quality. Make sure to read reviews on your favorite review website (like cnet.com) before buying.

Here are two models to illustrate the contrasting features and prices.

GPS Model	Features and Cost
Garmin eTrex Venture HC	Included maps: Highways and bodies of water. Battery life: 15 hours Memory: 24 MB Navigation: Buttons and joystick Cost: $130

GPS Model	Features and Cost
Garmin Oregon 400t GPS	Included maps: Highways and bodies of water.
	Battery life: 16 hours
	Memory: Expandable. Base stores up to 1000 waypoints and 50 routes
	Navigation: Touch screen.
	Other: Can share data wirelessly with other similar units.
	Cost: $500

The above description probably doesn't do justice to how slick the Garmin Oregon is, but it does illustrate that the basic features of location and mapping are available to the novice user at a reasonable cost. I didn't see anything in the more expensive models that would enable a nicer walk. Again, read some reviews before buying. Don't just buy a more expensive model because it costs more. You might just be paying for some obscure features you would never use.

JUST THE FACTS

How does GPS work?

The GPS system consists of 24 satellites circling the earth. At any time of the day at least 4 of these satellites are visible (i.e. have line-of-sight to the earth's surface).

Your handheld GPS receiver locates at least 3 satellites, determines your distance from each satellite, and then uses a mathematical formula to determine your location on the planet's surface.

This information is translated into your latitude and longitude and is then overlaid atop a graphical map.

Cars

There are a number of relatively new automotive technologies that directly benefit the senior community. For example, satellite radio keeps the savvy traveler well connected to music and news as they cross what was previously a signal-void "radio hell." And anti-lock brakes keep us all from skidding out on ice or gravel. These technologies benefit everyone, so we won't spend time analyzing them in this book.

But there is one new automotive technology that really helps the senior community more than any other—the onboard GPS.

The automotive GPS provides the driver with real-time verbal instructions on how to get to her destination. No more pulling over into the gas station to buy six maps and collect conflicting directions from a dozen different travelers who are probably as lost as you. Now you just program your destination into the GPS, the GPS determines your current location based on readings from multiple satellites, and then it calculates the best route to your destination.

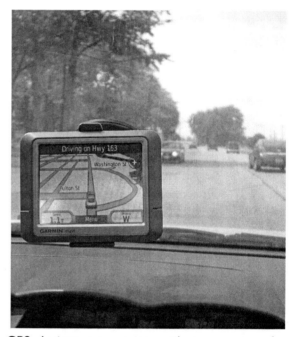

GPS devices can mount easily to your car for easy viewing while driving. I recommend, however, getting one that reads to you so you don't have to look at it.

Sure, sometimes (very rarely) the GPS will give you strange or incorrect information. But the beauty is that if it does, it is not your fault. You didn't get lost—the machine did! It will eventually correct itself and find the destination and you'll have the peace of mind that you didn't screw up. Brilliant!

Here are some features that you should look for in your onboard GPS.

✓ **Text to Speech.** Have the GPS receiver speak the directions to you. It's a lot easier to turn left onto Pearl street in 100 feet, when you hear a voice say, "turn left onto Pearl street in 100 feet." Driving and reading at the same time is usually not a great idea.

✓ **Pre-loaded maps.** Unlike the handheld hiking GPS devices, many automotive devices come with a complete set of road maps—not just the highways.

The range of GPS products is impressive—spanning prices from $150 to over $600. Here are a few well-reviewed GPS devices for a quick comparison.

GPS Model	Comments	Cost
TomTom ONE 125 - GPS receiver	Good no-bells-and-whistles entry level GPS system. Includes maps of the U.S and will speak generic instructions. Does not include text-to-speech, so will not include spoken street names.	$150
Magellan Maestro 4370	Quality GPS device with preloaded maps of U.S., Canada, and Puerto Rico. Includes text-to-speech function. Also features more complex route calculations, which can factor in real-time traffic updates (for a fee). Also includes a multimedia player to play music and video.	$400
Garmin Nuvi 880	Excellent GPS device that features an accurate voice recognition system. Push a button, speak your destination, and let the GPS tell you how to get there. This device also integrates nicely with Windows software—you can plan your route on your computer and upload to the GPS device. Additionally, you can get access to MSN Direct services like weather, traffic and stock quotes.	$550

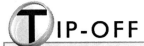

TIP-OFF

It's cold outside—the kind of cold that sinks into your bones and won't be warmed by a hot cup of Joe. The only thing colder than the temperature outside is the temperature **inside** your car. Brrrr! Imagine grabbing hold of that five-degree-below-zero steering wheel. Imagine the icy cold of the driver's seat pushing into your once warm flesh. Yuck!

There is a way to avoid getting into a cold car—the remote start.

You can install a device in your car that will allow you to start it from several hundred feet away. These devices are usually integrated with an electric keychain that will also unlock doors and pop the trunk. Some fancy models even allow you to control the temperature inside the car.

These devices range in price from less than $50 to more than $200. Oh… you should also pay for installation, which will run another one to two-hundred bucks.

Do you need this? No. Do you want this? Probably—especially if you have cold winters.

Search for "remote car start" on any search engine to begin your investigation.

Maps!

If you are resisting the GPS revolution, but still need to know where you are going, fear not! There is another mapping technology available to you.

Gone are the days of purchasing volumes of detailed maps for the different cities and states you plan to visit. Also gone are the days you need to call the restaurant and ask them for directions to their location. Now you view maps and print directions for free over the Internet.

A few of the big names in online maps are Mapquest (www.mapquest.com), Yahoo! (maps.yahoo.com), and Google (maps.google.com).

These free online mapping services allow you to:

✓ View detailed street maps of any city in the U.S.

✓ Retrieve and print driving directions between two points.

✓   View points of interest, stores, and restaurants around a chosen location.

These are just the basic features that nearly all map services provide. There are a few companies—most notably Google—who have gone above and beyond these basic mapping services to provide mapping experiences that are actually fun to just look at.

Let's investigate a few of Google's mapping innovations.

Satellite View

Google was the first map provider that included the option to see the satellite (or aerial) view of your map. Now you can search for your own address and zoom in to see an actual satellite photo of your house. You probably won't want to navigate using the satellite photos, but they are fun to look at.

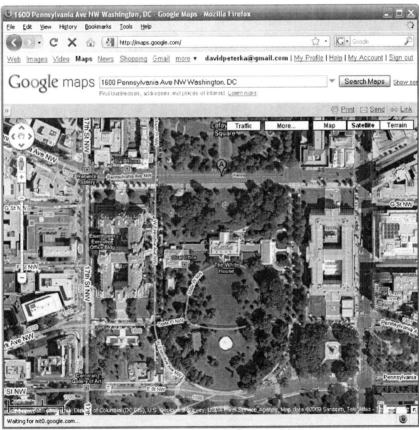

Satellite view of the White House using Google Maps.

Street View

You can now view a picture of the actual street for the location on the map. This option isn't available everywhere, but a large number of metro and suburban areas do have surprisingly good coverage.

Before your next trip downtown, try it out. Search Google maps for the restaurant you'll be patronizing, zoom in, and click Street View. Use your mouse to drag the picture to get a 360 degree view of the street. You'll be amazed at the quality of the photos.

Some people—for example, people who live in the apartments or houses being photographed—don't like this feature because they feel it's an invasion of their privacy. It may be, but it's still really slick.

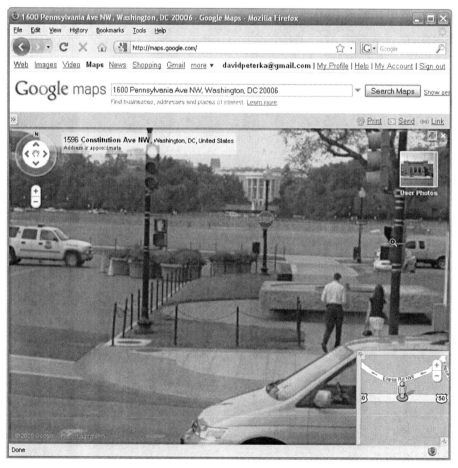

Street view of White House (in distance) using Google Maps.

Traffic

Google also allows you to display traffic statuses for most metro areas. Let's say you want to meet your daughter for dinner in downtown Chicago. It's nearing rush hour and you're not sure which route to take. You can simply look up Chicago, Illinois on Google maps and click the Traffic button. There you will see a traffic status for the city's major highways. Green means traffic is flowing freely. Red means traffic is slow or stopped.

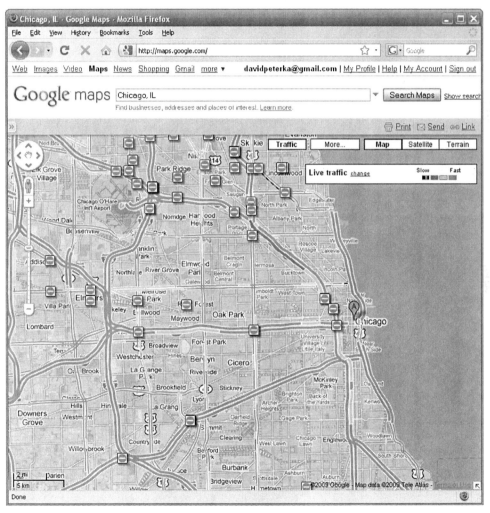

Live traffic view of Chicago using Google Maps.

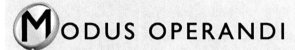

MODUS OPERANDI

How to print directions from Atlanta to Orlando using Google Maps.

Printing directions from point A to point B has never been easier. Here's how to find and print directions from Atlanta to Orlando.

1. Open a Web browser (like Internet Explorer).

2. Enter `maps.google.com` in the Web address field and click **Enter**.

   The Google Maps page opens.

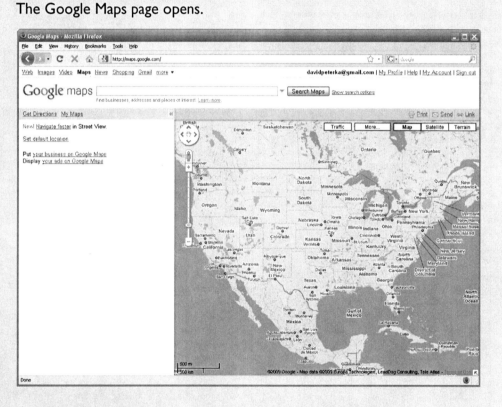

3. Click the `Get Directions` link in the upper left hand corner.

   Two fields, A and B, appear.

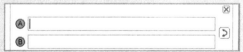

4. Enter Atlanta, GA in field A and enter Orlando, FL in field B.

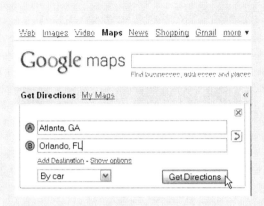

5. Click the **Get Directions** button.

Text directions are shown on the left and high-level graphical (map) directions are shown on the right.

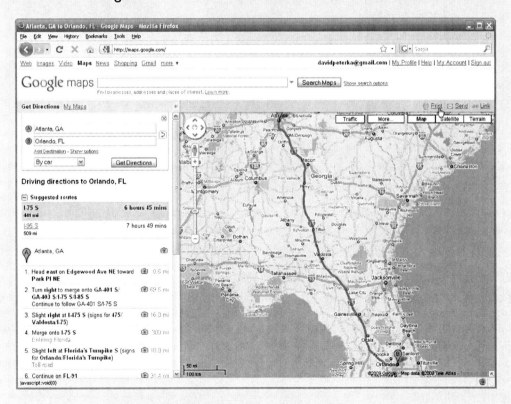

6. Above the graphical map, click the <u>Print</u> link.

A nicely-formatted print view opens.

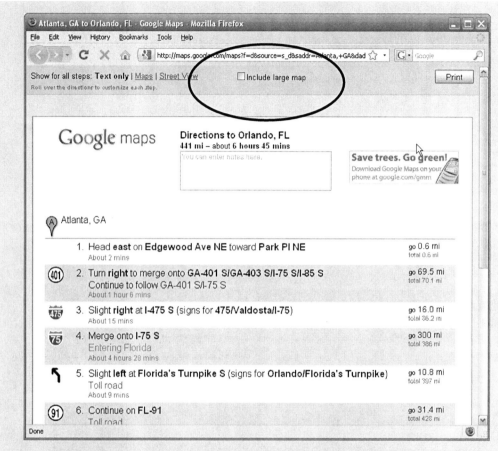

7. Optionally select the box at the top of the page to **Include large map**.

    This will print the graphical map along with your text directions. I always select this option.

8. Click the **Print** button in the upper right hand corner to print the directions.

    This will bring up your browser's print window.

9. Select your printer and click **OK** to print the directions.

    Remember that you need to be somehow connected to an actual printer—either physically through a plug or over a wireless network connection.

Google Earth

Google also offers a free interactive mapping product called Google Earth. This application provides global map and terrain information with a snazzy navigation. You can literally fly over Paris and swoop down to the Eiffel Tower to see a slightly squashed 3-D image. Zoom in more to get access to hundreds of photos from different vantage points.

But although the interface is a little slicker, this isn't that different than the satellite and street views from Google maps. There are, however, a few Google Earth features that make it worth the download:

✓ Google Sky—view the constellations from any point on Earth.

✓ Google Ocean—explore the Earth's terrain below the ocean.

✓ Historical Data—view cities and towns as they looked in the past (going back a few decades).

You'll need to download either the full application to your computer or the browser plug-in to get Google Earth running on your computer. You'll also need high-speed Internet to take full advantage of this nifty software.

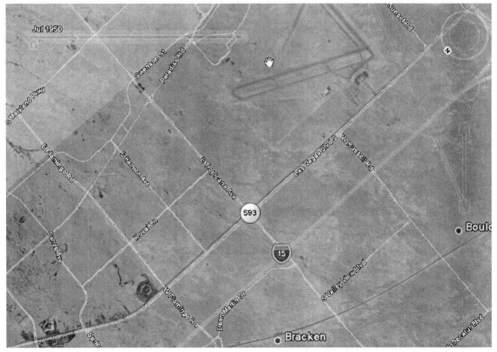

Google Earth picture of comparatively barren Las Vegas in 1950.

Futuristic Fun

We've entered a new millennium and transportation doesn't seem that different from 100 years ago. So where is your flying car? What about the Star Trek transporter machines to beam us from one place to another?

I have good news and bad news. The good news is that some of these futuristic technologies are close to reality. The bad news is that most remain economically unfeasible and appear not to have a marketable future in the near term.

Let's quickly investigate a few of these fun futuristic modes of transportation.

Jetpack

Believe it or not, you can already buy a jetpack.

But I don't recommend it.

The modern jetpack flies using a compressed gas or by an exothermic reaction such as hydrogen peroxide reacting with silver. The gas or steam rushes out of the pack and propels the wearer upward.

Awesome! Right? Well...

Flight times for the current jetpacks are hovering (no pun intended) just under a minute. And the actual flight apparatus weighs about 100 pounds. Oh, and did I mention that a jetpack costs between $100,000 and $200,000? Not exactly the most senior-friendly technology.

A few new jetpack models are scheduled to hit the shelves in 2010. One model claims it will use jet fuel to enable a 19 minute flight. Better, but still probably not worth several hundred thousand dollars.

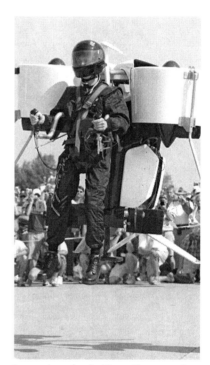

Jetpacks fun? Yes. For a few minutes. After that, you'd better be near the ground.

Flying Cars (Street-Legal Aircraft)

Since you have a few hundred thousand dollars lying around, I recommend skipping the jetpack and buying a street-legal aircraft. A few companies claim that these will be widely available by 2011.

One company, Terrafugia, has already built a prototype personal aircraft with retractable wings that can also be driven on any road. In street mode, the Terrafugia Transition gets 30 miles per gallon. In flight mode, you can travel more than 400 miles at speeds up to 110 miles per hour. It may look a little strange on the road, but it flies!

The company claims that these vehicles will be commercially available by 2012 with a sticker price of $200,000—which seems like a bargain when you consider it's the same price as a short-flight jetpack.

All you need to drive the vehicle is a standard driver's license. To fly it, however, you'll need a "sport pilot" license, which requires roughly 20 hours of training.

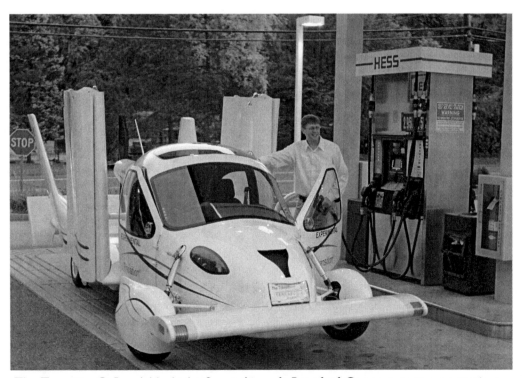

The Transition® Roadable Light Sport Aircraft Proof of Concept runs on premium unleaded auto gas. Carl Dietrich, CEO/CTO is shown with the Transition®.

There are other companies developing these street-legal aircraft, each with radically different designs. One looks like a dune buggy with a parachute. Another looks like a flying saucer. They will all be expensive. But they will also probably all be really interesting and fun.

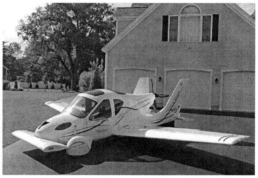

The Transition® Roadable Light Sport Aircraft Proof of Concept with wings extended at home.

Teleportation

Beam me up?

Scientists can do some amazing things. For example, they can obtain funding for projects investigating teleportation. More amazingly, they have made some progress!

Scientists have successfully transported photons (little pieces of light) from one place through space to another place. In these experiments, the particles are only teleported a few meters, but it's still amazing.

So when can we expect to see a full human teleportation device like we see on TV?

Probably never.

CLUE

Web Research
Visit the howstuffworks website for a really nifty explanation of how tele-portation may someday work.

In order to teleport a piece of matter you need to fully understand its quantum state—know EXACTLY how the thing is put together. This means that to transport a human, we would need a computer to analyze each of the trillion trillion atoms in the body and send that data to another computer where the human could be reconstructed with absolute precision. If any of your pieces/parts are slightly out of place, you could end up with severe mental or physical problems.

So, if I were you, I would hold off on teleporting anywhere for a while.

Home Entertainment

All work and no play make for a very boring person. Even the most dedicated Senior Sleuth should put down the magnifying glass now and then to cut loose.

Fortunately, there is no reason for seniors to stop playing or enjoying life. In fact, there are a number of technologies developed specifically to engage senior creativity and to entertain for countless hours. Television, movies, music, photography, games—these technologies are slicker than ever and provide thousands of hours of pleasurable life-enriching opportunities.

Of course there is junk programming out there—bad TV shows, boring games, and atrocious music. Fortunately, home entertainment technologies include excellent search features to help you filter out the bad and quickly find the good.

Technology has also opened up a new universe of user-created content. Now you can snap your own photos or produce your own videos and share them with the world.

With these fancy home entertainment technologies, you will never again utter the words, "I'm bored."

Chapter 8

In this chapter you will investigate:

➤ Television

➤ Music

➤ Digital Cameras

➤ Digital Video

➤ Video Games

➤ Electronic Books

Background Check

Home entertainment has received a technological makeover in the last century. Television programming has exploded and games have moved from the kitchen table to the computer console. Additionally, a few popular (and formerly technically complex) home-based hobbies such as photography have opened up to anyone with a computer and the itch to get creative.

Below is a high-level timeline of some major milestones in home entertainment technology.

1890

1895
Alexander Stepanovich Popov built his first radio receiver

1900
First use of word "television" at the World's Fair in Paris.

1901
Marconi picks up the first transatlantic radio signal

1904
Fleming invents the vacuum diode

1906
On Christmas Eve engineering professor Reginald Fessenden transmits a voice and music program in Massachusetts that is picked up as far away as Virginia.

1920
First scheduled commercial radio program.

1930
The first TV commercial is broadcast. The BBC begins regular TV transmissions.

1933
Edwin Howard Armstrong develops frequency modulation, or FM, radio as a solution to the AM static problem.

1940
Peter Goldmark invents a 343 lines of resolution color television system.

1947
Transistor is invented

1948
Cable television is introduced in Pennsylvania as a means of bringing television to rural areas.

1956
Ampex creates the first practical videotape system.
Robert Adler creates the first practical remote control.

1962
AT&T launches first satellite to carry TV broadcasts.

1964
Development of magnetic audio cassette.

1973
First video game, Pong.

1975
Texas Instruments develops first filmless camera. It was never sold.

1976
Sony introduces betamax, the first home video recorder.

1977
Nintendo sells its first TV console video game.

1979
First Walkman portable radio/cassette player released.

1986
Super VHS introduced.

1990
First commercially available digital camera. Release of Photoshop, software to digitally alter pictures.

1991
Kodak ships its first digital SLR camera for $13,000

1994
Playstation launches its game console.

1996
DVD video format introduced.

1997
Camera ships with megapixel resolution.

1998
First mp3 (digital music) player.

1999
First TIVO (digital video recorder) released.

2001
First iPod released.
Microsoft gets into the video game race with the XBOX.

2005
Playstation first to reach the 100 million unit sales mark.

2006
Wii launches with new wireless controller.

2007
Hulu.com launches website to provide streaming TV through the Internet.

2010

Television

There's nothing tricky about television. You plug it in and watch your shows. Right?

Well... no.

The simplest television configuration accepts signals over the air and then converts them into picture and sound on your TV. But if you're only using the signals captured by your antennae, then you are missing out on the wonders of cable and satellite television programming.

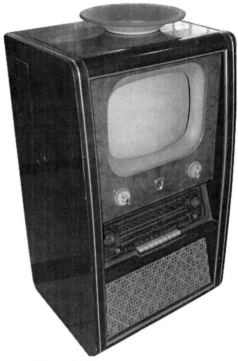

Not only do you need to consider the source of your TV signal, you also need to think about the picture quality. Do you want a high definition picture? Are you happy with your 27-inch screen or should you upgrade to the 48-inch flat screen plasma? And then comes the question of recording your favorite shows. Are you still using a VCR? If so, there are new recording technologies to consider.

Classic TV!
(Photo courtesy of Stefan Kühn.)

Let's investigate some TV technological developments.

Digital Signal Conversion

By now you should have converted your television to receive and display digital (rather than analog) signals. The U.S. Congress mandated that all television stations broadcast only digital signals by June 2009. This frees up a number of frequencies that can then be used by emergency teams (fire and police) as well as additional commercial wireless services.

If you had an old TV, then you needed to purchase an analog-to-digital converter to get your TV to work. If you've bought a new TV in the last year, then it almost certainly was shipped with a new digital tuner.

All of this is old news and you have probably already navigated through the FCC's techno-jargon to a reasonable solution for yourself. I only mention it for the rare case of someone who has that older television in their basement that they plug in only once a year for the "It's a Wonderful Life" marathon. Unless you have a digital tuner, George Bailey isn't coming around this year.

Flat Panel Revolution

Many people retire into a smaller home because they are easier to maintain and usually less expensive. But just because your house might have gotten a little smaller doesn't mean that your television has to. In fact, with the introduction of the flat panel television, you can get a monstrously-sized TV and hang it on your wall, thus preserving cherished floor space.

Just a few years ago, flat panel TVs were prohibitively expensive. But now you can get large screens with beautiful pictures for only slightly more than their boxy predecessors. It all comes down to supply overrunning demand while manufacturing materials and processes become less expensive. The bottom line is this—if you need a new TV, there is little reason to consider anything but a flat panel.

Flat panel televisions come in two technological flavors:

✓ Plasma

✓ LCD

Both of these technologies produce good pictures in a thin television. There are, however, a few differences worth noting.

Plasma

Plasma television screens include a matrix of small gas-filled cells that produce a picture when given an electric charge.

Advantages of Plasma:

✚ The picture colors tend to be richer and brighter, with a noticeably deeper black.

✚ Wider viewing angle. If sitting to the side of an LCD television, the colors can appear distorted.

LCD

LCD television screens hold liquid crystals sandwiched between two sheets of glass that produce images when given different electric charges.

Advantages of LCD:

+ Less power to operate than Plasma equivalent.

+ Lighter than plasmas and therefore easier to wall-mount. (This is really only a concern if you plan on mounting the TV yourself.)

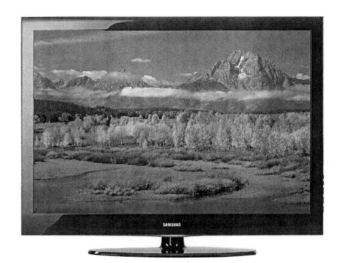

42" Samsung LCD TV, which at a glance looks just like a Plasma. Differences between LCD and Plasma are in picture color and quality.

+ Can be used at high-altitude. The gas in plasma TVs will expand in the lower pressure at high altitude and will distort the picture. If you're moving to the Alps, then take your LCD.

+ Not subject to picture "burn-in," which can leave a ghost image on the screen in some plasma models.

Plasma or LCD—The Verdict

Although I have listed more advantages for the LCD models, I'm not sure there is a clear winner here. You can get roughly the same quality television (screen size and resolution) for comparable costs. And the color differences are barely noticeable to the casual observer.

If you are an artist and your eye is trained to appreciate and scrutinize color, then you'd probably be better off with a plasma TV. If you live above 6,500 feet, then you must purchase an LCD TV. Otherwise, I would just wait until you found a good deal on either, check out the picture quality in a showroom, and get it.

Both technologies are fantastic and you'll never regret purchasing either.

The ~~Blasted~~ Blessed Remote

We love them and hate them.

We love them when they work and hate
them when they don't. And if you're new to
a particular remote, then it might seem like
the thing is not working more often than it
is working. Let's say you accidentally bump a
button to shift the remote into DVD controller
mode. Then you can push (or smash) your
buttons until you are blue in the thumb and it
won't change the blasted channel.

Remote controls are often complicated by the
thing that makes them so powerful—their ability
to control multiple devices. Because they can
do everything, you often find that they are too
complicated for you to do anything with them.

Let's take a look at a few remote control options.

A Different Remote Control for Every Device

This is the most straight-forward remote
operation. Each gadget hooked up to your
TV will have a separate remote control, with
the product name prominently displayed on
it. For example, the Samsung remote goes to
the Samsung DVD player, the Sony remote
to the Sony plasma television, and the cable
TV provider will have their own cable remote.
Simply use the remote for the activity you want.
To turn on the TV, press power on the TV
remote. To navigate through the cable channels,
use the cable remote.

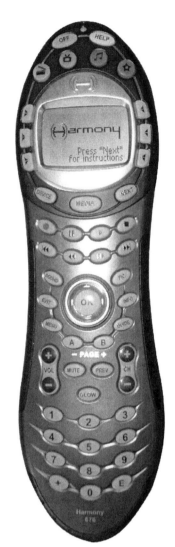

Remote controls can be
quite complex.

Of course, the cable remote will likely have a
feature to allow you to control your TV's power
and volume. But you don't have to use that feature. If you want, you can
keep all of your remote controls device-specific. Then all you have to do is to
find an end table big enough to hold all of them.

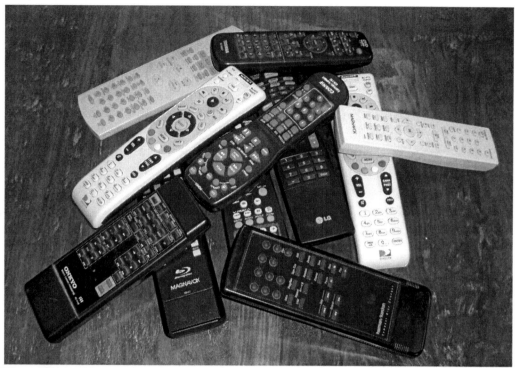

The coffee table can be consumed with too many remotes for too many electronic systems.

Universal Remote

A universal remote is any remote control that can control multiple devices. The low-end universal remotes only allow you to control a small list of devices set by the manufacturer. Your Cable or Satellite TV is an example of a device that will control multiple devices—your cable box and your TV (for most new TV models). The high-end universal remotes can be hooked up to your computer and updated to interface with all of the latest devices (TVs, DVDs, and DVRs) as they come onto the market.

Although some universal remote interfaces are navigable by the novice user, the high-end devices are really marketed towards the techno-crazy

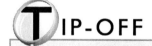

TIP-OFF

Many cable and satellite providers will give you a remote that will likely integrate with your television set. This will allow you to turn on the TV, adjust the volume and change channels with one remote control.

user. These people enjoy creating macros (small programs that run a series of commands) for their remotes.

Setting up a universal remote to interface with multiple devices can be a hair-pulling experience. It usually involves slogging through onscreen menus and entering a series of multi-digit numbers representing the other devices to incorporate. Some companies have heard this complaint and have addressed it. For example, the Logitech Harmony One allows you to connect the device to the computer and then answer a series of easy-to-understand questions. At the end of the process, your remote will control just about anything you could imagine hooking up to your TV.

Universal remotes range from $30 to $300, with the high-end devices hovering around $250.

Large Button Remotes

Big buttons can make a big difference. There are now a number of large-button universal remotes designed to allow people with arthritis or vision impairments to operate multiple devices from one controller. To be honest, these things look a little silly—a little like old-fashioned adding machines. But what you sacrifice in style you make up for in accessibility and comfort.

Here are two examples of large button universal remotes.

Tek Partner Large Button Universal Remote

This remote (shown on the right) features big keys for easy access and is shaped like an I for easier grasping. You can use it to control up to 4 devices. It costs around $40.

Big Button Universal Remote Control

This remote also features large keys. In addition, it includes lighted keys for easier viewing. Like the Tek Partner, this can control up to 4 devices. It costs around $25.

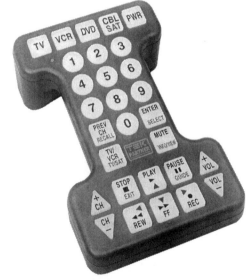

Tek Partner Remote—one option for senior remotes.

Recording the TV

Remember the VCR? You may as well forget it. There are now better ways to record your favorite programs.

Now you can purchase a Digital Video Recorder (DVR) to record only the shows you want. Yes, I know. This sounds like what a VCR does, but trust me—DVRs are better.

Here's why:

✓ DVRs record programs on a digital hard drive, so you no longer need video tapes.

✓ DVRs have higher picture and sound quality than VCRs.

✓ Many DVRs include advance programming features so that they will repeatedly record the shows you like. In fact, many devices can learn the types of shows you prefer and then recommend other similar shows that you would probably enjoy.

✓ Many DVRs have a lovely interface that makes recording programs easy.

Most cable and satellite TV providers now provide a DVR add-on option. Depending on the company, they may charge you for

TIP-OFF

TIVO is cool.

TIVO pioneered digital video recording and still holds a special place in the heart of avid consumers. TIVO boasts more features than cable and satellite DVRs (such as optional wireless support and online scheduling), but it will probably cost you a little more—at least up front. TiVo requires that you purchase (not lease) their DVR device, which runs between $150 and $600 depending on the model. Monthly service costs are similar to cable and satellite providers.

More expensive models generally mean more storage capacity at a higher resolution. The least expensive model records 80 hours of standard (not high-definition) TV where as the most expensive model stores up to 150 hours of HDTV or 1,350 hours of standard resolution.

the equipment, but it's more common that they just include the equipment in the monthly subscription fee. In fact, many DVRs are integrated with the receiver, so you don't even need an extra box sitting by your TV. Ignoring any additional equipment charges, DVR service will cost you around $10 per month above your normal television service.

TV on the Internet

Let's say you're taking an RV trip across the county. Because you are a technology junkie, your RV is equipped with the latest and greatest satellite Internet access. You can check your email, review online maps of surrounding areas, find instructions for changing your spark plugs, and, most importantly, watch your favorite television programs.

Broadcast companies have struggled with the problem of how to deliver content over the Internet. If everyone were downloading programs from the Internet, then the advertisers would be less interested in paying for the TV commercial spots.

Broadcasters' first response was to sue anyone who posted a copyrighted program on the Internet. This turned out to be impractical because too many people were doing it. (It turns out that we are a nation of technological law breakers.) Somewhat reluctantly, broadcasters fell back to the old adage, "if you can't beat them, join them."

Broadcasters now offer their content through "streaming" media. Streaming means that you must be connected to the Internet to watch the program (i.e., you cannot download the

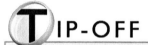

TIP-OFF

Netflix Website

If you prefer movies to television programming, then there is a nifty website you should check out—www.netflix.com.

This site allows you to create a queue of DVDs you would like to watch. These movies are then mailed to you as they become available. Different subscription levels allow you to check out a different numbers of DVDs simultaneously. For example, the cheapest subscription allows you to have only one DVD at a time.

If you rent even a few movies each month, the subscription ends up being cheaper than renting through your local video store.

Netflix also offers streaming movies, although their selection is more limited than their huge mail-order offering.

program to your machine and then watch it later—or share it with your friends). This allows the broadcasters to include advertising, which was previously stripped from the programs by the content thieves (or pirates).

Many broadcast companies (ABC, CBS, and NBC) post full episodes of their latest shows as streaming media on their websites. You'll have to download a different plug-in for your browser for each company in order to watch their shows.

A better choice for watching TV online is through a company called Hulu (www.hulu.com). They post the last five episodes of many popular shows, so if you missed one, then you can easily get caught up. Their web interface is nice, streaming is reliable, and the quality is good. Hulu specializes in online program delivery and so beats the other broadcast companies who specialize in creating content (like ABC and NBC) hands down.

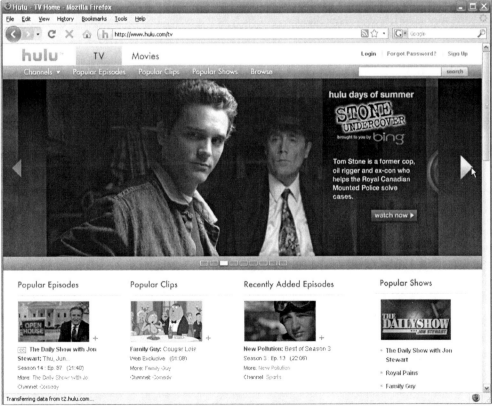

www.hulu.com is a great website for watching TV online.

Music

Music technology has trended in three directions—smaller, smaller, and smaller.

This is great news for the Senior Sleuth. Now you can inconspicuously listen to inspiring music while on your next investigation. Just grab your MP3 player, stick the small (nearly invisible) speakers into your ears, and you've got your own thrilling soundtrack! Depending on your musical tastes, this could make your stakeouts much more enjoyable.

Sound quality has also improved with the move to digital music. Music is no longer produced on large vinyl records or magnetic tapes, which tend to deteriorate over time, producing that old scratchy background sound. Now it's all CD (compact disc), downloadable MP3 (small computer file), or streaming media from the Internet. Music sounds sharper and doesn't deteriorate with time.

The net result is that you can now take your favorite music with you wherever you go. Yes, of course, we've had Walkmans for decades, but these required you to bring briefcases full of tape cassettes. As we get older, we want our luggage to get smaller. These new music technologies help.

MP3 Players

MP3 players are the digital successors to Walkmans—portable music players using either tape cassette or DVD music storage. Instead of storing your music on tapes or CDs, MP3 players store music on their miniature computer-like hard drives. Whereas one cassette tape held one album's worth of music, a moderately-sized MP3 player can hold 30 albums of high-quality digital music. Of course, larger capacity models can hold much more music than that and many can even store and display videos.

MP3 players consist of four components:

✓ **MP3 player body.** The mini-computer that stores musical data and provides all sorts of playback options.

TIP-OFF

If you plan on listening to your music through a home entertainment system, you can still go the MP3 route. The easiest way to do this is to plug your MP3 player into your stereo IN plug.

✓ **Headphones.** The small or large device you wear in or over your ears to hear the music.

✓ **Computer connection.** A cable or docking station that connects your MP3 player to the computer for the purpose of uploading your music onto your player.

✓ **Music (MP3) files.** Digital music files, obtained (usually) from the Internet and uploaded from your computer.

You can convert your existing music into MP3s and then load them onto your player. You can also purchase new albums or individual songs already in the correct digital format from online music stores.

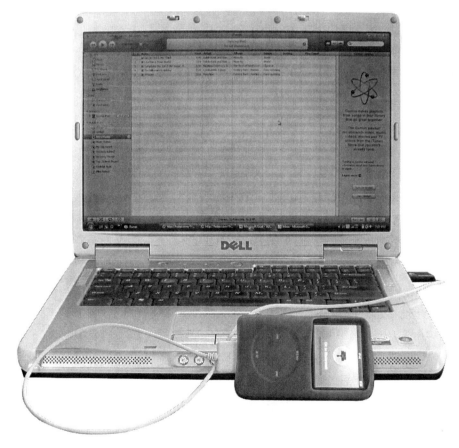

MP3 player connects to computer for music synchronization and battery charge.

iPod

Apple's iPod is the reigning king of MP3 music players. In fact, people will often use the term "iPod" to describe any MP3 player regardless of manufacturer.

iPod is the name of the product line, which includes a number of different models. The current product line includes:

iPod Shuffle ($80)

Tiny MP3 player that can either play music sequentially or at random (shuffled). The Shuffle does not include a screen where you can select individual songs.

iPod Nano ($150)

Thin, light, small player with a screen and click wheel (consisting of only four buttons and nifty scroll feature) used to select songs.

iPod Classic($250)

Slightly larger player with a bigger display and more storage. Features the fabulous click wheel. The larger display makes video viewing more enjoyable.

iPod Touch ($229)

MP3 player delivered with a nifty touch-screen interface for watching videos, playing games, taking and viewing photos, sending email, and browsing the web. This is essentially the iPhone device without the phone.

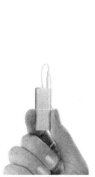
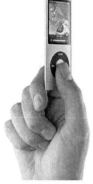
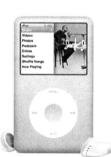
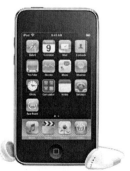

iPod Shuffle   iPod Nano   iPod Classic   iPod Touch

Other MP3 Players

There are dozens of companies manufacturing MP3 players, and there are hundreds of models that are less expensive than the iPod devices. Depending on your use, these models may provide an excellent value for you.

Here's a small sampling of companies putting out quality MP3 products: Sony, SanDisk, RCA, Finis, Samsung, Creative Zen, Insignia, and Microsoft.

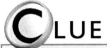

CLUE

MP3 Players

Read reviews on the MP3 player before you buy. If there is a problem with the quality, the reviews will tell you. If the model doesn't work for your use pattern (for example, you like to swim with your music) then it's better to find out before you buy.

MODUS OPERANDI

How to purchase a song for your MP3 player (overview).

You can buy single songs or entire albums from a number of websites. Two of the most popular music sites are Apple's iTunes (www.apple.com/itunes) and Amazon.com. Here's an overview of the process.

1. Purchase the song.

    a. Visit an online music retailer: for example, Amazon.com.

    b. Search for a song, artist or album that you want to purchase. For this example, look for The Beatles' song "Yellow Submarine."

    c. Gasp as you see there are 71 songs with this title. Luckily, each result lists the artist, so you can pick the Beatles' version rather than some tribute band.

    d. Listen to a short preview of the song to make sure you're buying what you think you're buying. You want the original recording, not a live version.

    e. Click the **Buy** button and proceed through checkout where you enter payment information such as credit card info, shipping info and billing address. Note: It's OK to put your credit card information into a trusted (and secure) website like Amazon.

    f. Save the MP3 to your computer.

2. Upload the song to your MP3 player. You should follow the instructions provided with your MP3 player. But here's a summary of the process.

    a. Connect your MP3 player to your computer. Your player came with a special cord that will fit into a slot on your computer or laptop. It will probably fit into the USB slot.

    b. Open the MP3 software that came with your player.

    c. Locate the file on your computer and move it to your MP3 player.

    d. Disconnect the player.

3. Enjoy the music!

TIP-OFF

You can get music onto your iPod by installing and running iTunes—Apple's music store and management software. iTunes will automatically catalogue all MP3 files on your machine and add them to your music library. You can then select to upload any files in your library onto your iPod. See `store.apple.com/ipod` for more information on these nifty gadgets.

Online Music

Are you sick of your music library? Want to hear something new? Then your first thought is probably the radio. Before you go adjusting your tuner, why not try exploring new music online?

There are two flavors of online music:

✓ **Radio stations that stream their broadcasts.** Listen to the radio broadcast through your Internet connection. There are literally thousands of radio stations to choose from. These stations tend to play either popular contemporary songs or hits from the oldies. With this option, you take what they give you.

✓ **Smart Internet music delivery.** Select your favorite artists and musical styles and allow the website to recommend songs that you might enjoy. You can then interact with your musical selection—rating songs as good or bad—and the website will tailor the music to your tastes.

Of the two options, I recommend experimenting with the "smart Internet music delivery." Try a website like www.pandora.com. After you create an account, you can select an artist that you like and Pandora will create a "radio station" with artists and songs of similar style to your selection. Select multiple artists to include in your "Quick Mix" and be entertained for hours, days, or weeks with music you are guaranteed to enjoy.

MODUS OPERANDI

How to create a Pandora music station.

You can create a music station based on just one artist. Pandora will then locate and play other similar artists.

1. Open a Web browser (like Internet Explorer).

2. Enter www.pandora.com in the Web address field and click **Enter**.

    The Pandora home page opens.

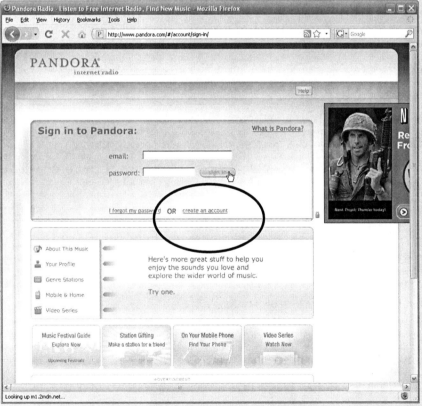

3. Click the create an account link.

    The Register for Free page opens.

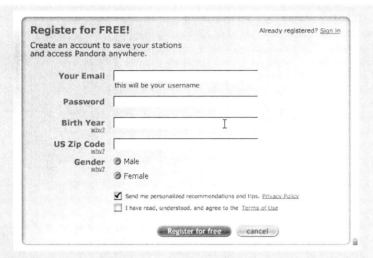

4. Enter your email, a password, birth year, zip code and gender.

    Pandora requires this information for data trend tracking. They want to know who's listening so they can share this generic information with advertisers. Don't worry, though. Pandora will not sell your personal information to telemarketing companies.

5. Check the box for `I have read, understood, and agree to the Terms of Use.`

6. Click the **Register for free** button.

    Your account is created and a new advertisement page opens.

7. Click the **No Thanks** button at the bottom of the page to skip the ad.

8. If presented with another option to enter your email password, optionally click the **skip for now** button.

    A new page opens where you can search for an artist to create your radio station.

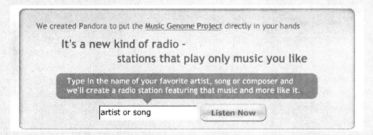

9. Enter the name of an artist and click the **Listen Now** button.

10. Pandora locates your artist and begins playing music that you should (at least in theory) enjoy!

Converting Your Music to MP3s

Now that you're moving to digital MP3s, what do you do with all those boxes full of old Sinatra albums? Or the thirty love-song-filled mix tapes you made for your wife for your 20th anniversary? Or the 200 CDs you bought because everyone said that they were the media of the future that would last longer than a cockroach after a nuclear war?

Simple.

Convert them to MP3s.

The process differs slightly depending on the music format. CDs are the easiest to convert—requiring a simple software program on your computer. Tapes and vinyl are a little trickier—requiring some additional hardware.

Converting CDs

If you have a relatively new computer and operating system (Windows XP or Vista), then you can use Windows Media Player to "rip" your CDs into MP3 files. Just insert a CD into your CD/DVD drive, open Windows Media Player, and select the **Rip** button at the top of the player. The software will do the rest—prompting you for any additional actions you might need to perform.

The MP3 files will be created on your computer as specified in the Rip tab's "More Options" settings. You can then import them into your MP3 player software and then upload them to your player.

There are a number of CD ripping software programs available for sale, but I don't see why you actually pay for them. When given the choice, go for free.

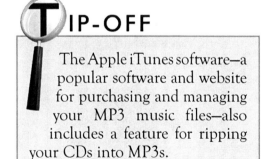

TIP-OFF

The Apple iTunes software—a popular software and website for purchasing and managing your MP3 music files—also includes a feature for ripping your CDs into MP3s.

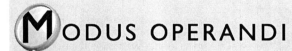

MODUS OPERANDI

How to "rip" a CD to MP3s using Windows Media Player.

The process for converting music from your CD into an MP3 is called "ripping." Here's an easy way to rip your old CDs into MP3s for use on your MP3 player.

1. Insert a music CD into the CD drive on your computer.

   If you are using Windows XP or Vista, then the following window opens.

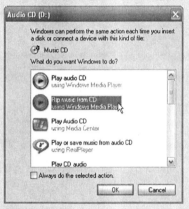

2. Click on **Rip music from CD**.

3. Click **OK**.

Windows Media Player opens to the Rip window and begins converting your CD to individual MP3 files. The files are stored in your Windows Media Player Library.

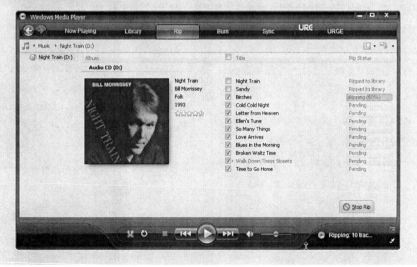

4. And you are done!

The music files are now located on your computer. By default, files are located in the following location `C:\Documents and Settings\[account name]\My Documents\My Music`.

You can listen to the newly ripped tracks by clicking on Library tab at the top of Windows Media Player and searching for the artist or album.

Converting Tapes and Vinyl

Assuming that you have a turntable and tape player, then all you need is one more gadget to convert your tape cassettes and records into MP3s. You need a special part that connects your stereo to your computer.

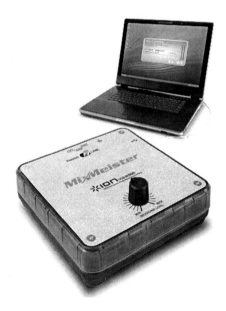

There is a nifty gadget out there, which also includes a software package for easy ripping—Ion's U Record. This little box comes with RCA cables for connecting to your stereo and a USB cable for connecting to your computer. Plug everything together, run the included software on your computer, and play your tape and records to rip them into MP3 files.

U Record product links your stereo to your computer so you can convert your tapes and vinyl to digital (MP3) music.

This product is available at most stores that sell electronics, including Target, Radio Shack, and Circuit City. It costs around $50, a small price to pay to have all of your favorite recordings digitized.

Digital Cameras

We've seen hundreds of film-based cameras over the last century—from large format view finders to disposable underwater cameras. You snapped some pictures and then sent the film off to some lab where they charged you to develop and print a few copies. If you were really photo savvy, you built a darkroom in your spare bathroom and developed the pictures yourself—tweaking the composition and cropping with your own artistic discretion. But more likely, you just sent the film away and hoped that they came back with at least a few good pictures.

In summary, photography of the past was expensive, slow, and forced you to print all pictures good and bad.

This all changed with digital cameras. Digital cameras:

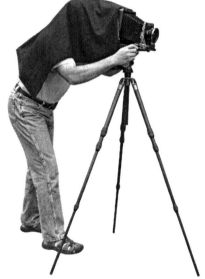

✓ Do not require film.

✓ Display your pictures on a small viewing screen.

✓ Allow you to delete really bad shots.

✓ Do not require developing.

Snap your pictures, optionally use a software program to digitally alter color and composition, and then print from a home photo printer.

Classic large format view camera. Modern digital cameras are much, much, much smaller.

If you don't have a photo printer, you can print selected pictures (the good ones) by uploading them to an online printing service, such as www.snapfish.com, who will print and then mail the photos to you quickly for a very reasonable cost. Or you can upload the digital pictures to your local Walgreens over the Internet. They'll print the pictures and you can go to the store and pick them up.

Digital cameras allow for instant gratification. Go to a party and snap a few pictures of your friend Herbert talking to the floor plant after consuming one too many drinks. The next day you can email the digital photo to all of your friends and family. Go ahead. Herbert will think it's funny.

Digital Camera Features

When shopping for a digital camera, you'll want to pick a camera with the features that match your photo style. If you plan on snapping pictures inconspicuously at family gatherings, you would use a different camera than if you were photographing Half Dome at Yosemite National Park.

Here are a few features you should consider when buying a digital camera:

✓ **Resolution.** Camera resolution determines the maximum print size of your picture. Most cameras now are shipping with more than 6 megapixels, which will allow a larger print than you would ever want. The higher the resolution, the more options you'll have for cropping and still getting a good print. The more expensive cameras will always have higher resolution.

✓ **Memory.** Most digital cameras store their pictures on small memory cards that are inserted into the camera. You can have multiple cards or just one high-capacity card. A one-Gigabyte card will store around 800 pictures— more than enough for any party or vacation. Remember that you can always delete the bad pictures on the fly.

✓ **Video.** The quality isn't usually that great, but you can take short videos using many digital cameras. Sometimes you need more than a still shot of your grandkid eating his chocolate birthday cake. Sometimes you need to see the whole gooey process.

WATCH IT!

Never put a camera in your checked luggage—it will be destroyed. Mine was.

✓ **Size.** As with all modern electronics, cameras are trending smaller. You can get a camera that fits in the palm of your hand, but you might need to sacrifice picture quality, features, and camera usability. It's hard to hold some of those little cameras.

✓ **SLR and Lenses.** SLRs are the high-end camera for the photo enthusiast. These cameras often allow you to attach different lenses for different photo options—close-up portraits versus long-range wildlife photography. SLRs resemble the nicer 35 millimeter cameras of yore. These cameras also differ from other digital cameras in that you look through a small viewfinder (rather than a digital display) when taking your pictures. You can later review your photos on a display.

Photo Printers

If you find yourself printing one-off pictures for friends and family, you should consider getting a photo printer. Photo printers are specially-marketed inkjet printers (as opposed to laser printers). They will give you the flexibility to print, view, tweak, and print again to get a final picture that is truly pleasing (at least to you).

Your first thought is probably, "Fantastic! I can now print all of my pictures for free. No more uploading my files to some weird website. No more trips to Walgreens to pick up my photos." Your first thought is, sadly, wrong. It actually costs more to print pictures at home.

Here's a quick cost breakdown for home printing.

Color Inkjet Printer Example: HP Photosmart A636	$100
Ink Cartridges (300 pages of color)	$30 (or $.10/page)
Photo Paper (100 sheets of 4x6 glossy paper)	$12 (or $.12/picture)

So even ignoring the price of the printer, you would still pay around 22 cents per print. The same sized 4 x 6 photo prints at Walgreens cost between 12 and 20 cents per print.

Printing pictures through an online retailer is almost always cheaper. But printing at home is more immediate and can produce better results. Unless you are a photo enthusiast who must control photo color output completely, you'll probably be happier using the online photo printing websites.

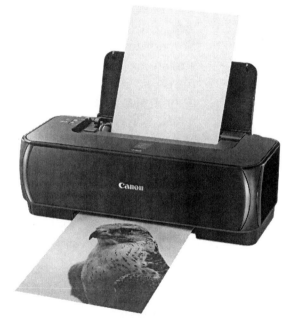

Photo printers can produce great prints from your own home... for a price.

MODUS OPERANDI

How to print a picture using the Snapfish Website.

You can upload digital pictures to the Snapfish website (and other websites) and then order prints, which you can hang on your wall or mail to friends and family. Here's how to do it.

1. Open a Web browser (like Internet Explorer).

2. Enter www.snapfish.com in the Web address field and click Enter.

    The Snapfish home page opens.

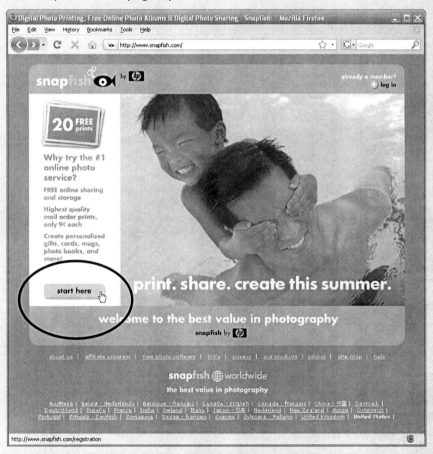

3. Click the **start here** button.

    The registration page opens.

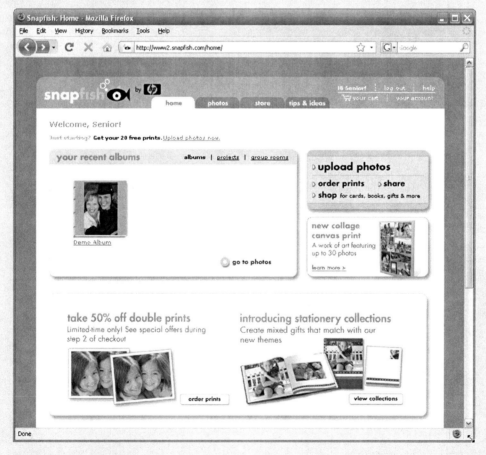

4. Enter your first name, last name, email address, and password.

5. Click the box for `I accept the Snapfish terms and conditions.`

   NOTE: At the time of this printing, a new user was offered 20 free prints. For this example, we'll skip the free offer so you can see the typical flow. Rather than accept the offer, I have clicked the link to proceed to my snapfish home page.

6. Click **Upload photos**.

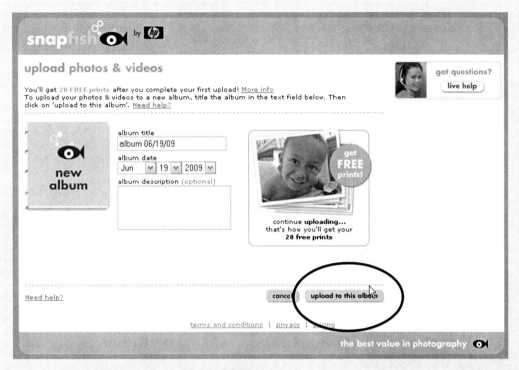

7. Enter an album title, date and description.

8. Click the **upload to this album** button.

    The `upload photos` page opens.

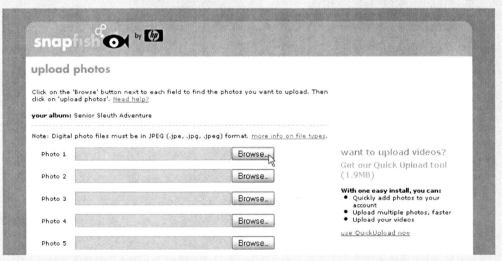

9. Click the **Browse** button to locate a digital photo to upload to your album.

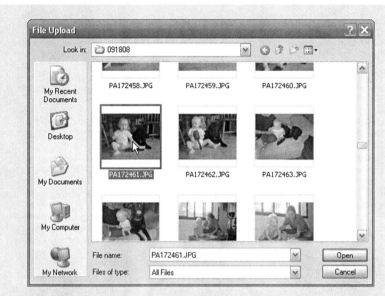

10. Locate and select a photo from your computer and click **Open**.

11. At the bottom of the upload photos page, click the **upload photos** button.

    Wait as your photo is uploaded to the snapfish website. This may take a few minutes.

12. When the photo upload completes, click the **view entire album** button.

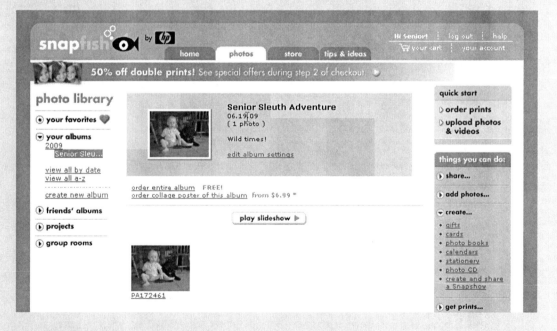

13. Click the picture you want to print.

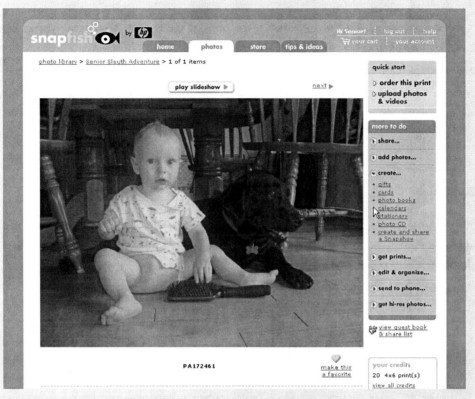

14. In the upper right-hand corner, click **order this print**.

    This places the picture in your shopping cart.

15. At the top of the page, click the your cart link.

    Your cart opens.

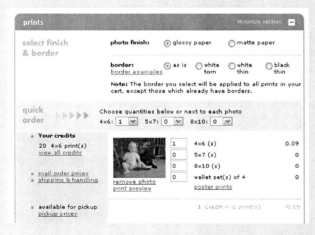

16. In the prints section, enter the number of prints (of each size) that you would like to print. For this example, I will print just one 4x6 print.

17. Click the **check out** button.

18. Complete the order by entering your shipping and billing information in the following pages.

Posting Photos Online

This is the digital age. You no longer have to print photos in order to share memories and events with friends and family. Now you can share pictures electronically onscreen.

There are two common ways to share photos electronically:

✓ **Email.** Attach the photo file to an email and send to whomever you like.

✓ **Post the photo on a website.** Upload the photo to any of a number of photo-sharing websites (like Google's Picasa site) or your social network site (like Facebook). Then send an email to your friends and family with a link to your online photo album, where they can see pictures and even leave comments.

Emails are great for sending one or two pictures, but you can't beat the free online photo websites for sharing lots and lots of pictures. Most of these sharing websites give the visitor the option of buying prints of a photo that you've posted. This, along with advertising, is how they make their money.

Here are a few online photo sharing websites. You'll need to create an account in order to upload photos and create online albums.

| www.kodakgallery.com | Provides "free" photo sharing. Kodak recently changed their photo hosting policy, and now they require you to purchase a minimum amount of photos each year to keep your pictures there. I only list this site because it's fairly popular. But you can do better by using one of the other free services. |

www.flickr.com	Provides truly free photo sharing. Also provides nifty tools for editing your photos (for example, getting rid of red-eye), organizing photos into albums, and purchasing printed cards and photo books.
picasa.google.com	Picasa offers similar features to Flickr, but in its slick Google way. The interface is great, organization tools are fantastic and editing features are easy to use.

Picasa is my preferred photo site, but you can't really go wrong with Flickr either. Hey, they're free. Why not try them both to see which you like better?

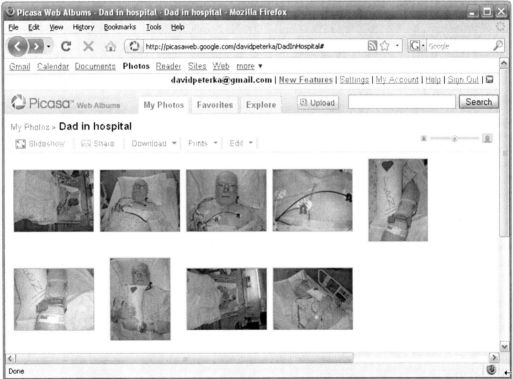

Post-surgery photos posted on the Picasa website. (The surgery went well, thank you!)

Modus Operandi

How to email a photo.

You can attach a photo to an email and send it to your friends. Here's how to do it using Google Mail.

1. Open a Web browser (like Internet Explorer).

2. Draft an email to one or more friends and family members. See Chapter 6 (Communication) for step-by-step instructions.

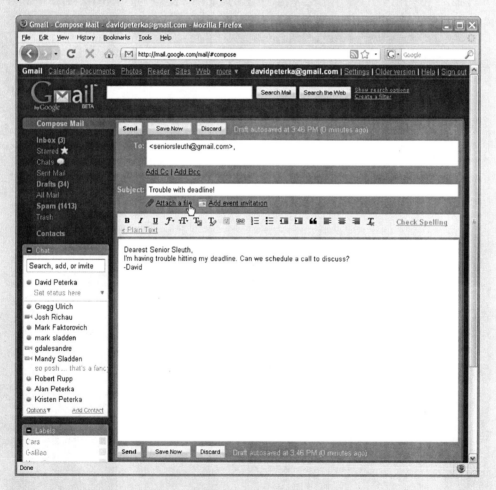

3. Beneath the Subject line, click `Attach a file` to locate a digital photo.

   A new window opens.

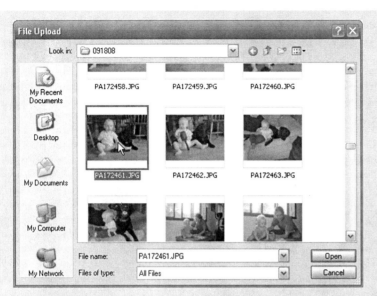

4. Locate and select a photo from your computer and click **Open**.

    The digital photo uploads to your Gmail account.

5. When the upload completes, click **Send** to send your email (and photo) to friends and family specified in the email's To field.

Editing Your Pictures

There are dozens of software programs for editing your digital photographs. Use these programs to resize, crop, edit coloring, or apply a host of other effects to your pictures. Some of these programs allow you to cut and paste objects from other photos and blend them seamlessly together. For example, if you don't like the way your hair (or lack of hair) looks in a photo, you can paste a picture of a hat onto your head. Problem solved.

The most popular (and most powerful) photo editing software today is Adobe Photoshop. There is nothing you can't do with Photoshop. In fact, the term "photoshop" has become synonymous with altering a digital picture. For example, someone might say, "there was an ugly guy in that picture, so I photoshopped myself out."

Photoshop is a complex program and will take some time to learn, but if you are a serious photographer, you may want to buy a copy. The current version costs $699 from Adobe's website. Yes, this is a lot of money, but it is the top-of-the-line photo editing software. You may be able to find older versions for sale for a lot less. In fact, I recommend it. The older versions are still jam-packed with more features than you'll ever need.

If, however, you are a casual photographer and are mostly satisfied with the way your pictures look unedited, then you can probably get by using a free editing software. I will again point you to the easy-to-use Google Picasa. Microsoft also ships a free Paint program that will allow you to edit, crop and perform minor tweaks to photos.

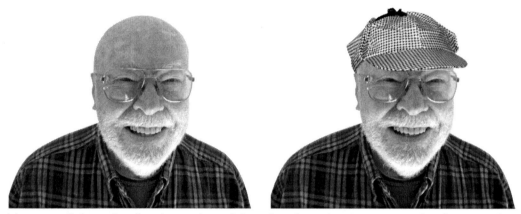

It's easy to "photoshop" a picture. It took less than five minutes to copy a hat from another picture onto this one.

Digital Video

Sometimes the low-resolution videos taken on your digital camera aren't good enough. Sometimes you want to zoom in on the action and take extended footage of kids and grandkids playing around the old swimming hole. For these occasions you'll need to get a digital video camera.

There are hundreds of video cameras on the market. Some are small enough to fit in the palm of your hand, others are so big that you need to hold it over your shoulder. Some require small magnetic tapes or DVDs to store the video, others store data in the camera on internal hard drives. Some are loaded with professional features, some are not.

With all of these options, purchasing a video camera can seem a daunting task. But don't get too stressed out. That's not the Senior Sleuth way. After considering a few basic options and reading a few hundred reviews, you'll be filming the next great American home video.

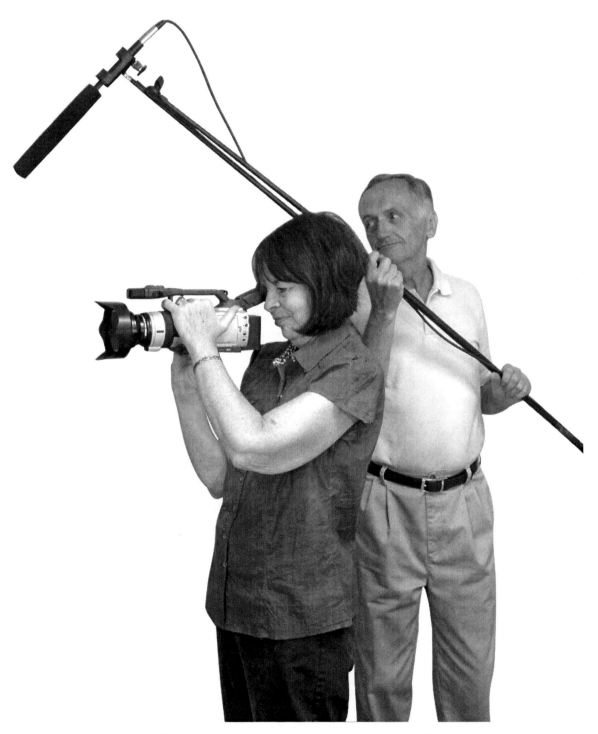

The Senior Sleuth video crew recording a nefarious crime!

Digital Video Camera Features

Modern video cameras are jam packed with hundreds of features that you will probably never use. With that said, there are a few camera features that you should consider when shopping.

Media Storage

Different cameras store their video data on different media. Here are the most common:

Mini DV tapes Small magnetic tapes that store your video digitally.	Advantages: Good quality. Disadvantages: Requires multiple tapes; slow transfer to computer for editing or publishing (most download in real-time, so 60 minutes of video requires 60 minutes to transfer).
Small DVDs Mini DVD discs loaded into your camera.	Advantages: Easy playback on most DVD players. Disadvantages: Low recording times (30 or 60 minutes) with average quality.
Flash Memory Tiny memory cards similar to the ones used in digital cameras.	Advantages: Smallest, most compact media leads to super-tiny cameras. Disadvantages: Short recording times.
Hard Disks Spinning disk permanently inside the camera, similar to the hard drive on your computer.	Advantages: Easiest download to computer for editing. Disadvantages: Hard disk can skip if performing extreme activities while filming.

High Definition (HD)

HD video cameras record video at high definition for a crisper display on HD televisions. These camcorders are more expensive and require more storage space for the videos. This means you'll need a bigger, better computer to edit the video.

Optical versus Digital Zoom

Optical (meaning lens-based) zoom captures better close-ups than digital zoom. Digital zoom basically enlarges the video picture, resulting in pixilation and blurring when digitally zooming too close. If you're looking to zoom in on action at a distance (for example, filming wildlife), you'll want a camera with a good optical zoom (at lease 10x zoom).

Note that many camcorders have both optical and digital zoom, with the digital zoom taking over where optical stops.

Image stabilization

The camera can digitally smooth out the video as you shoot. This comes in handy for people with shaky hands or who are moving while taping.

TIP-OFF

Should you buy an HD video camera?

As of this printing, I wouldn't recommend it. HD cameras are more expensive and most of us only watch our home videos once a year. If, however, you plan to take more serious videos (for example, your grandkids' weddings), then you could opt for the HD camera. Picture quality will generally be better—especially when viewed on your HD television set.

Digital Video Cameras—User Profiles

When buying a digital video camera, consider how you intend to use it. Are you going to record the occasional grandkid's soccer game? Take it on your next international adventure? Produce a series of thirty-minute documentaries on your secret life as a Senior Sleuth? With realistic expectations on your usage, you can quickly narrow down the list of appropriate cameras.

Home and Vacation Movies

Small, light, inexpensive.

This is the best camera profile for shooting short movies around the house or on your next vacation. You want a small and light camera to fit into your carry-on luggage. And you want an inexpensive camera because 1) you are not a Rockefeller, and 2) cameras can take a beating during even the most tranquil vacation. I've already dropped two into the ocean.

Here are two well-reviewed models that meet this profile.

Kodak Zx1 HD Pocket Video Camera (black)	Storage: 2 GB flash (not expandable) Size (inches): 2 x 0.8 x 3.9 Weight: 3.3 ounces Cost: $160 Best Used For: Short video clips that you intend to upload directly to the Internet. With a short zoom (2x), this is not a good choice for filming wildlife.
Canon FS11	Storage: 16 GB Flash (expandable) Size: 2.3 x 4.9 x 2.4 Weight: 9.2 ounces Zoom: 37x optical; 2000x digital Cost: $350 Best Used For: Casual taping of friends and family. The video quality falls in line with the budget price, but unless you plan on distributing your videos to network television stations, it's probably OK.

Remember that there are dozens of camcorders in this price range, with a host of features and designs that you might find attractive.

Just one more thing...

Some of these super-compact camcorders may prove difficult to operate. In order to fit everything on the device, controls are small and often doubled up. For example, your camcorder may have a scroll-wheel (for moving through camera menus) that you can also click to make selections. This is why you must go to a store to inspect these products before buying them. I usually research my top three choices

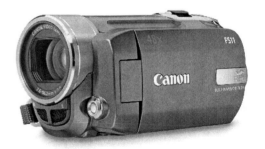

Tiny Canon FS11 video camera for home movies.

online, go to a store to try them out, and then buy the device online (where you will almost always get a better deal).

Filming Formal Events for Friends and Family

Let's say that your neighbor's grandkid is getting married and she has asked you to videotape the wedding. "No pressure," they tell you. "It doesn't have to be professional. We just want to get the I do's and first kiss."

You've been waiting for an excuse to get that new camcorder, and now you have it!

But which camcorder should you get?

The two top requirements must be—and forgive me if this is obvious—sound and picture. You want something good, relatively small, but you don't want to spend $1000 dollars. And because love is forever (insert small cynical wink here) you might want to consider upgrading to a high-definition camcorder to future-proof your purchase.

Here are a few models to consider. All of these are high-definition cameras and allow you to attach a separate external microphone. Remember to check reviews and similar models before you buy.

TIP-OFF

Microphones

If filming a formal event, consider using a directional, or shotgun, microphone to focus in on the sound that you want without picking up ambient noise to your sides or back.

Canon Vixia HV30	Storage: Mini DV tapes
	Size (inches): 3.5 x 5.4 x 3.2
	Weight: 1.2 pounds
	Zoom: 10x optical; 200x digital
	Cost: $600 and up.
	Best Used For: High quality home videos. Remember that you'll need to buy the mini DV storage tapes for all of your videos. These aren't expensive, but costs add up.

Canon Vixia HG20	Storage: 60 GB hard disk
	Size: 3.1 x 5.4 x 3
	Weight: 16.4 ounces
	Zoom: 12x optical; 200x digital
	Cost: $600 and up
	Best Used For: High quality home videos. Hard disk storage makes for easier computer uploads and eliminates need for purchasing additional tapes.
Sony Handycam HDR-SR11	Storage: 60 GB hard disk
	Size: 3.3 x 5.4 x 3
	Weight: 1.2 pounds
	Zoom: 12x optical; 150x digital
	Cost: $975 and up
	Best Used For: High quality home videos. Excellent picture and good audio.

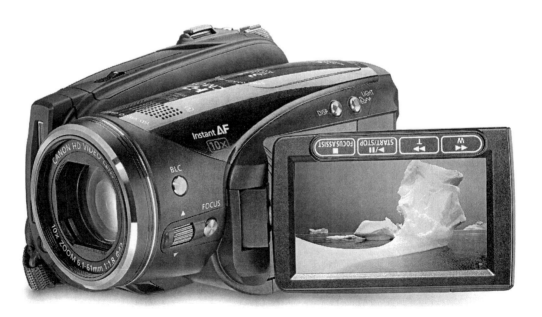

Canon Vixia HV30

Professional Videographer

Sometimes you need the very best. If you are planning on filming and broadcasting an independent film or documentary, you'll need a professional camera like the one listed below.

Canon XH A1	Storage: Mini DV tapes.
	Size (inches): 6.4 x 13.8 x 7.4
	Weight: 4.7 pounds
	Zoom: 20x optical
	Cost: $2,800 and up
	Best Used For: Professional video—independent films, documentaries, etc. These cameras are much larger than the small consumer video camcorders. If filming long sequences, I recommend investing in a good tripod.
	Note that this camera, though providing professional quality, does not film in HD.

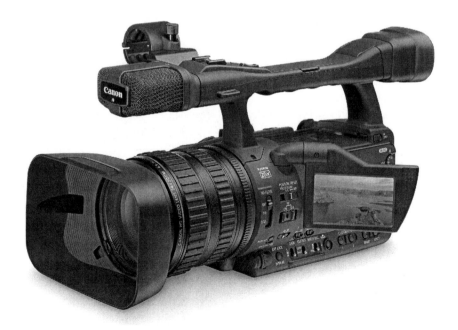

Canon XH A1 Professional Video Camera

Editing Digital Video

After filming the great American home video, you have three distribution choices:

✓ Dump the footage somewhere (a dark closet, perhaps) and forget you ever filmed the event

✓ Burn your raw footage to a DVD or post it on the Web

✓ Edit the raw footage into something coherent, sleek, and entertaining— and then post it.

I usually edit my videos. I end up re-watching them more often and am more inclined to allow friends and family to see them. Nothing fancy, mind you. I mostly just shorten the clips, add some transitions, include a few titles, and slap down a simple soundtrack.

But to accomplish even a simple editing job, you must have the correct software. Fortunately both Windows and Macs offer free simplified video editing software. If you're thinking of making video production a full-time passion, then you might want to upgrade to one of the more powerful (and more expensive) video editing programs.

Video Editing Software

If you just want to splice together some clips, include some basic effects, and slap down a limited number of simple audio tracks, then you can easily get away with using the free video editing software from Windows (Windows Movie Maker) or Mac (iMovie).

If, however, you want to include more complex audio and visual effects (like color matching or green screening), then you'll have to bite the bullet and buy video editing software. Here are a few to think about.

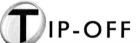

TIP-OFF

Free Video Editing Software
I strongly recommend trying the free video editing software that comes with your Windows or Mac computer before buying any of the above software. You may find that they have all of the editing features that you'll ever need. You might also decide that the free programs are lacking some critical feature (at least, critical to you) that you are only aware of because you've tried editing video. You'll be able to make a more informed purchasing decision after playing around with the free versions.

Software	Features	Price
Professional-grade software Adobe Premiere Pro and Apple Final Cut for Mac	Professional video editing software programs. Adobe Premiere Pro works with Windows and Mac. Final Cut Pro works only with the Mac OS. High resolution editing. Flexible video capture (i.e., can import video from a lot of different cameras in a lot of different video formats). Features many, many more transitions and effects compared to the free or bargain editing software.	$799 (Premiere) $600 (Final Cut)
Bargain video editing software. Cyberlink PowerDirector Corel VideoStudio	These software programs provide good interface for capturing your video (i.e., uploading video to your computer), editing video on a timeline, adding simple effects and including a soundtrack. You get the same types of features as the professional software programs—you just get fewer of them. But unless you are going to be editing a lot of effects-rich video, these programs will likely provide all of the features you need.	$120 (PowerDirector) $80 (VideoStudio)

MODUS OPERANDI

How to edit a video—an overview.

Here's the high-level process for how to edit a short video. Note that you can find lots of free video tutorials online that provide a lot more detail. Search for "how to edit a video" on www.youtube.com for a bunch of examples.

1. Download the video footage from your camera to your computer. Note that you'll need a lot of disk space. Video files are huge. Refer to your video camera user's guide for instructions.

2. Open your video editing software—for example, Windows Movie Player.

3. Import the video clips into the video workspace.

4. Drag and drop clips to the timeline.

5. Trim the clips so they fit nicely together.

6. Adjust the volume for the clips.

7. Add a music track.

8. Add titles and text.

9. Preview your movie.

10. Publish to CD, DVD, or the Web. (See discussion below.)

Publishing Digital Video to DVD and the Web

All video editing software programs include features for publishing video to either a DVD or to the Internet. You'll need to read the directions for your specific software, but here's the general procedure. I'll use Windows Movie Maker for illustrative purposes.

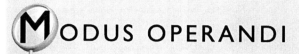

MODUS OPERANDI

How to publish a video to a DVD.

The following process assumes that you have a DVD drive capable of recording DVDs in your computer.

1. Insert a blank DVD into your computer's DVD drive.

2. Click **Start > All Programs > Windows Movie Maker** to launch Windows Movie Maker.

3. Open your video project (which you have already edited).

   a. Select **File > Open Project** from the menu.

   b. Navigate to your movie and select it.

   c. Click **Open**.

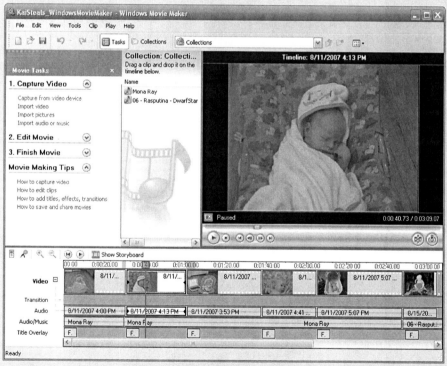

4. Select **File > Save Movie File** from the menu.

   The Save Movie Wizard window opens.

5. Click on **DVD**.

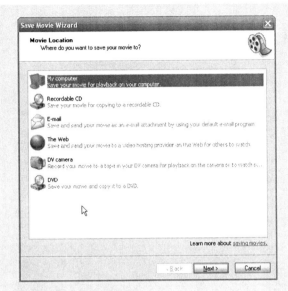

6. Click **Next**.

    The movie takes several minutes to save. The Create a DVD window opens.

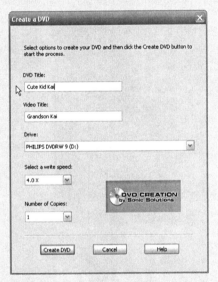

7. Enter a DVD Title and Video Title and click the **Create DVD** button.

When the DVD is done "burning," take it out of your computer, plop it into your DVD player, and watch your creation on the TV screen.

MODUS OPERANDI

How to publish a video to the YouTube website.

The easier way to share videos is by posting them on a website. The most popular of all video websites is YouTube (www.youtube.com).

You'll need a YouTube account to post videos. Go to www.youtube.com and click the Create an Account link. It'll take about 3 minutes and then you can post videos to your heart's content.

To post a video to the web (again, I'll use Windows Movie Maker for an example):

1. Open your video editing software.

2. Open your video project.

   a. Select **File > Open Project** from the menu.

   b. Navigate to your movie and select it.

   c. Click **Open**.

3. Select **File > Save Movie File** from the menu.

   The Save Movie Wizard window opens.

4. Click **My Computer**.

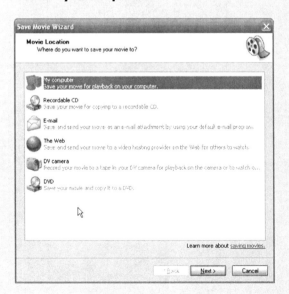

This is slightly non-intuitive. You would think that you should select The Web, but that's a little trickier. The easiest way to upload a video to You Tube is by starting with the movie file on your computer.

5. Click **Next**.

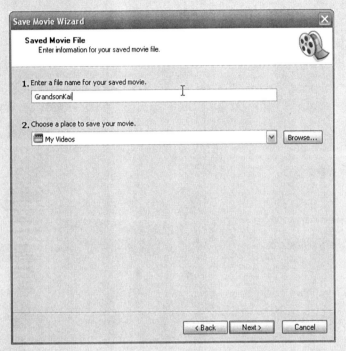

6. Enter a name for your movie and select where to save the movie file.

    You can accept the default location. Just note where it is so you can find the file later.

7. Click **Next**.

8. Select **Best quality for playback** on my computer.

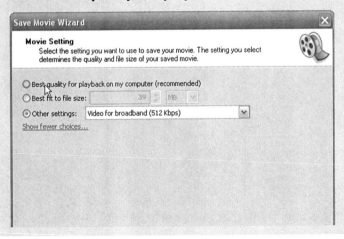

9. Click **Next**.

The file saves to your computer.

10. Click **Finish** to close the computer window.

11. Upload the file to YouTube.

    a. Go to `www.youtube.com`.

    b. Click the `Sign in` link (top right) and log onto YouTube with your user account.

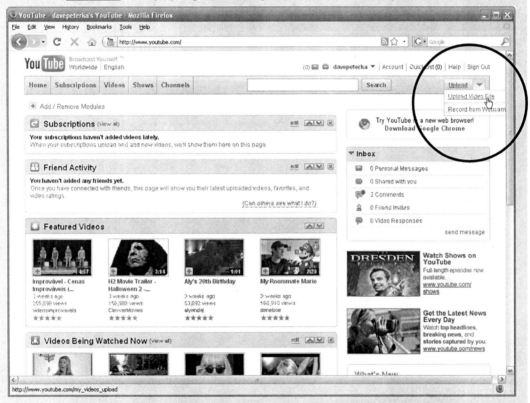

    c. In the upper right hand corner of the page, select **Upload > Upload Video File**.

      The Video File Upload page opens.

Video File Upload

Press "Upload Video" to select and upload a video file.   [Upload Video]

    d. Click the **Upload Video** button.

      The Select file window opens.

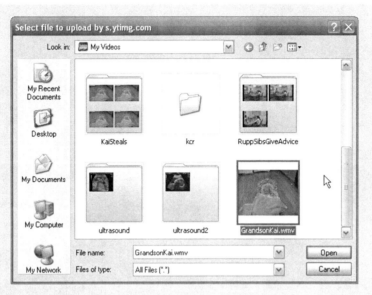

e.   Locate and select the movie file created above.

f.   Click **Open**.

The video file uploads to YouTube.

g.   Click the `Go To My Videos` link to see the newly posted video.

h.   Click on the new video to view the video.

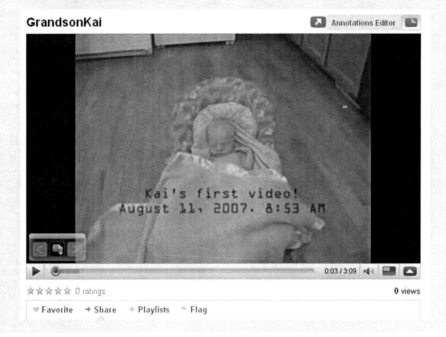

You can share the video with any friends and family with an email address. Below the newly posted video, click the <u>Share</u> link to see a variety of email and sharing options. For example, you could copy the provided web address (URL) into an email, or you could click the Facebook link to post the video on your wall.

Video Games

Video games are not just for kids. And I'm not talking about the brain-games that are designed to sharpen the aging brain and stave off Alzheimer's. I'm talking about normal video games that both young and old play for entertainment.

There are far too many individual video game titles out there to list them all, so we'll focus our investigation on the following topics:

✓ **Popular video game systems.** A summary of the main players and products in the video game market.

✓ **Video game categories.** Types of games from racing games to puzzles.

✓ **The Nintendo Wii.** A unique game system that is taking the senior community by storm.

I don't expect you to run out and buy each of these systems, but maybe the quick descriptions here will give you some insight into a grandkid's recreational terminology. On the other hand, don't rule out buying a system for yourself. There are plenty of games that

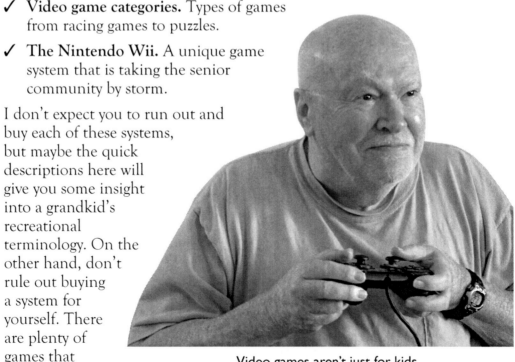

Video games aren't just for kids.

can offer hours of entertainment and social stimuli. Chances are you'll find a few that you enjoy.

Popular Video Game Systems

Here's a rundown of the most popular video game systems.

Game System	Highlights	Cost
Sony Playstation 3	Nice easy-to-use interface with quiet operation. WiFi interface with the Internet. Media player can play music and features a nice photo album for viewing photos. Includes a Blu-ray DVD player for viewing high definition DVDs. This is the only console that can play high-definition movies.	$399
Microsoft Xbox 360	Includes a hard drive to store your games for a better (faster and quieter) experience. Models with larger hard drives cost more. Hooks up to the Internet (via cable) to download game demos before buying them. This is really nice! Media player can display your pictures and play your music. Great Dolby Digital Sound. Includes a DVD player. Currently features more popular games than the Playstation 3, but this could change.	$299 and up
Nintendo DS Lite	Handheld video game device. Features fun games on a tiny device. Great for travel.	$130

Game System	Highlights	Cost
Sony PSP 3000	Playstation's handheld video device. Similar to the Nintendo DS, but with better graphics, and the ability to play videos and music.	$199
Nintendo Wii	Nifty game system that features a unique wireless controller that can sense your motion. This system is very popular among seniors.	$250
PC	You can, of course, still purchase video games for your PC. Some games are graphics-intensive, and will require special video hardware to properly operate.	You already have a computer, so this is essentially a free console.

Most video games cost between $30 and $60. Some are less, some are more. You can usually purchase video games for a deep discount from stores that sell used games. One of your first stops should be Amazon.com to see if there are any used copies of the game you want.

Video Game Categories

There is a video game for everyone. Do you like solving geometric puzzles? Or do you prefer gunning down hordes of alien invaders? Either way, you're in luck.

Here's a quick summary of the most popular video game categories.

✓ **Arcade.** Classic game category which gained popularity in the 1980s. These are typically two-dimensional games where you evade attacks or solve single-screen puzzles. A few examples are Pacman, Qbert, and Tetris.

✓ **Role Playing.** You play a single character who walks around and interacts with other computer characters. The other characters provide clues for your goals—often in exchange for your character's food or money. These games tend to have fantasy or science-fiction themes. They can take several weeks to complete. This is a popular category for PC games.

✓ **Strategy.** You control armies or other groups of people to obtain a goal. The goal could be to build a new civilization or wipe out an enemy. These games are fast-paced and demand intense multi-tasking. If you like the board game Risk and don't mind some heart-thumping pressure, you might like these games. This is a popular category for PC games.

✓ **Action.** Games where you run around blasting monsters, aliens, or other people to bits. These games tend to be very violent and visually gruesome. Unfortunately, this is one of the most popular game categories among kids.

✓ **Shooters.** Similar to the action category with lots of blood and guts flying around. Shooters feature a first-person view of the action. You can typically see your gun and blast anything in your field of vision. These are also very popular among the kids.

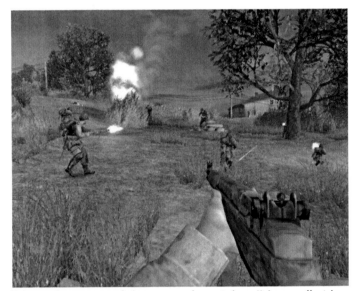

Picture from one of the many ultra-violent "shooter" video games. (Picture courtesy of Ubisoft.)

✓ **Driving.** Get in a car and race. Depending on the game, you can often select your car and race environment. For example, you could choose to race through San Francisco in a Pinto. Many racing games have multi-play where you can compete against your friends.

✓ **Sports.** Play football, soccer, hockey, baseball, and virtually any other sport. These games also tend to be multi-player games.

✓ **Puzzles.** Solve geometric puzzles, word puzzles, puzzles requiring careful dexterous movements, or brain teasing puzzles.

✓ **Exercise.** Popularized by the Nintendo Wii, you can now get a workout while playing video games.

Nintendo Wii (Pronounced "Wheee!!!")

The Nintendo Wii is a game system that features wireless remotes and motion sensors so that your movements control the character's onscreen movements. For example, if you're playing Wii tennis, you swing at the ball and your onscreen character also swings. Time it right and you'll actually hit the virtual ball!

Each Wii system ships with the Wii Sports game package, which allows you to play tennis, baseball, golf, bowling and boxing in front of your TV. No running is required—just hold the remote and swing at the ball (or opponent's face, if boxing) and the Wii players will mimic your action.

One of the most popular Wii games among seniors is bowling. In

TIP-OFF

Hold onto the Wii!
Make sure to wear the wrist strap when playing the Wii. Many TVs have been broken as the remote flew from the hand, across the room, and into the television screen.

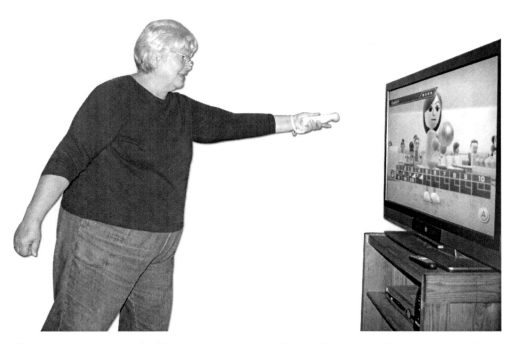

Characters are controlled by your movement. You make the bowling motion, and the character throws the ball.

fact, Wii bowling tournaments are becoming commonplace in retirement communities. Just hook the Wii up to that big screen TV, invite a bunch of friends over, get some pizza, and bowl! It's cheaper than bowling (after purchasing the Wii), easier on the back and doesn't require the funny-looking shoes (though you can still wear them if you'd like).

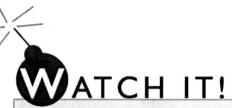

WATCH IT!

Make sure you clear any and all exercise routines with your doctor—even Wii fit.

The Wii features exhilarating games in a number of categories: sports, racing, arcade, role-playing, and puzzles. The Wii has also revolutionized the video game exercise experience with the Wii Fit product.

Wii Fit

The Wii Fit product features a series of exercises that the player performs on the Wii Balance Board. The Wii Balance Board is a low profile mat that detects your center of balance and weight. It then uses this information (along with the normal Wii motion sensor) to translate your movements to your onscreen character.

The exercises (games) include yoga, strength training, aerobics, and balance routines.

The player enters his age and height and Wii tracks his fitness. Certain exercises are only unlocked after you perform a number of qualifying exercises. In other words, this product is designed to get you in shape without killing you.

The Wii Fit bundle (balance board

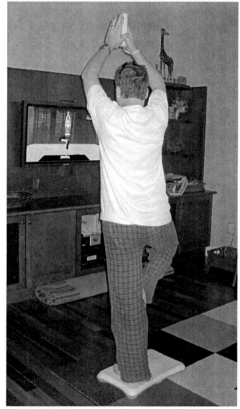

The Wii Fit games may be a good way to get a little exercise on a rainy day.

and software) costs around $90. Yes, if you have money sitting around, you're still probably better off joining a gym and paying for a personal trainer. But the Wii Fit is a fun alternative for that certain someone who wants a little extra exercise with low cost and funny, yet inspiring, graphics. If your kids or grandkids have the Wii Fit, try it out to see if it's a fit for you.

Electronic Books

Yes—books have gone electric. You can now purchase and download books to read on your computer or a special electronic reading device. But why would you? Great question, Senior Sleuth. Let's look at a few pros and cons of the electronic book.

Pros:

+ **Cheaper price per book.** New releases cost approximately $10 and older books are even cheaper. You can easily save $10 or more per book purchase. This can add up to huge savings—especially if you buy lots of new releases.

+ **Adjustable font size.** You don't have to seek out the large-print books. Simply adjust the font size on your electronic reader (or computer) and save your eyes from some unnecessary strain.

+ **Small and light reading devices.** You can read books on a small electronic reading device (like the Amazon Kindle). These are great for travel. Take a dozen books with you on your next beach vacation without having to haul around thousands of pages.

+ **Less printed paper is good for the environment.**

TIP-OFF

Download Books and Other Media to Your Kindle

Instead of lugging around a dozen books on your next vacation, simply download the books onto the Kindle. In fact, you don't even need to download the books before you leave. Using Kindle's wireless access, you can download a book from anywhere in the U.S. In addition to books, you can use Kindle to subscribe to magazines and newspapers and surf the Internet.

Cons:

- **You must have an electronic reader.** Sure, you could read these books on your computer screen, but that would not be pleasant. For an enjoyable reading experience, you'll need a specialized hand-held electronic reader, like the Amazon Kindle. These run about $300, but remember that if you buy a lot of new release books, you'll quickly recoup your investment by saving on the reduced electronic cover price.

- **Can't share.** When you love a book, you'll want to hand it to a friend so they can share in the literary experience. Well, you can't really do that with electronic books. The electronic files are non-transferable, so the only real way to share would be to lend someone your electronic reader. But then what would you use?

- **It's just not the same.** You don't get the same feel or smell of the book. No sound of flipping pages. No challenge of holding an 800 page book open with only thumb and pinkie strength and raw determination. You will miss these things—at least at first.

TIP-OFF

Which Reader?

At the time of this printing, the best electronic reader remains the Amazon Kindle. Sony did, however, just announce their upcoming reader the Daily Edition. In addition to wireless access, the Daily will feature a nifty touch screen.

The Sony reader will compete with the Kindle, but we'll have to see how it looks and feels before we know if it's a serious competitor. Initial pricing will be approximately $100 more than the Amazon Kindle.

So should you try it? I think so—especially if you buy a lot of books.

The price and ergonomic pros (in my opinion) outweigh the mostly nostalgic drawbacks. But before you run out and buy one, find a friend who has one and ask to borrow it for a week. Download your favorite book and give it a try. I think you'll be surprised with what a nice experience it is.

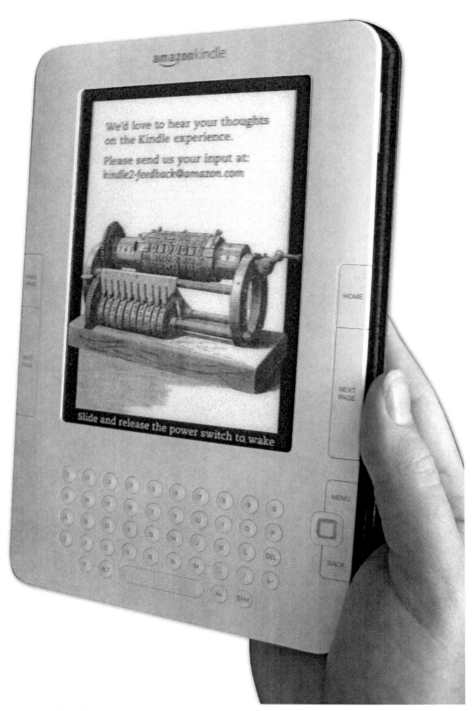

Amazon Kindle electronic book.

Futuristic Stuff

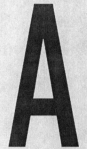

L et's grab our crystal ball and peer into the future. Actually, let's just do a little sleuthing on the Internet. The result will be the same—a glimpse at some stunning futuristic technologies.

Some of the following futuristic technologies are decades from realization, while other are already deep into the research and development stages.

Let's take a look at a few of the more interesting technologies, and then wildly speculate as to how these technologies could be beneficial to the senior.

In this appendix you will investigate:

➢ Quantum Computers

➢ Nanotechnology

➢ Humanoid Robots

Quantum Computers

Quantum computers are futuristic machines that will utilize the strange properties of quantum mechanics to perform calculations. At the heart of this idea is the concept of superposition. Whereas normal computers store information in bits, which can be either a 1 or a 0, a quantum computer stores its information in Quantum Bits (or qubits), which can be a 1, 0, or both! Yes, I know. It makes no sense at all, but this is what they tell us.

Superposition will allow computers to perform massive parallel processing. Using special algorithms designed for the unique quantum superposition quality, these computers will be able to solve math problems in seconds that would have taken normal computers a near infinite amount of time to solve. Pretty snazzy.

The most obvious application of the quantum computer is code breaking. So you can bet that governments around the world are watching this technology carefully.

The other application—which may more directly benefit seniors—would be in designing complex systems and materials. Imagine new lightweight materials in robotic limbs. Imagine small complex computers integrated with your clothing or attached directly into your brain. Imagine cities with stoplights that actually decrease congestion.

Far-fetched? Yeah, but not impossible (except maybe the stoplight bit). Many of our visions of the future rely on smaller and faster computing power. Quantum computers may hold the key to this future.

People have already performed simple quantum computer calculations, but there are still a number of technological challenges related to building the hardware. Some optimistic futurists put this technology in the hands of governments and big business within 10 years. More people lean toward 20 years.

Nanotechnology

Nanotechnology, often called nanotech, is an area of science and engineering dealing with tiny particles—on the atomic or molecular scale. This technology has the potential to impact every modern industry.

✓ **Industrial.** Nanoparticles can be combined with other standard materials to create new and useful properties. Need something as strong as steel but flexible as rubber? Nanotech may be the answer.

✓ **Health care.** Nanoparticles can be programmed to help repair tissue or rebuild failing organs. Or maybe you'll just take a pill (filled with nano-sized-robots) to unclog that pesky heart valve.

✓ **Communications.** Small communication devices could be included in our skull to wirelessly connect to other people or the Internet. Access all the world's knowledge with a single thought.

Nanotechnology is already here with more modest applications such as making a better sun screen. However, many experts say that society-changing breakthroughs (like the ones listed above) will start appearing as early as 2020.

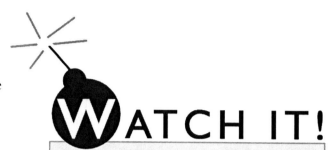

WATCH IT!

Nanotech does introduce a few environmental concerns. For example, if a particle is small enough to slip through the blood-brain barrier, we could see a host of unwanted injuries or neurological disorders. And how will nano-manufacturing impact our rivers and forests? The bad news is that nanotechnology could mean the end of life as we know it by introducing unexpected plagues and diseases. (Insert nervous laugh here.) On the flip side, people are watching out for this. And we're going to get some really slick products in the meantime.

Humanoid Robots

Sure, we have robots to sweep our floor and mow the lawn. But when will we get the real robots? If you're like me, then you can't wait for a mass market humanoid robot to clean up after you, walk your dog, and do your taxes.

Where is my robot butler?

The answer is: closer than you think. Maybe.

If you search the Internet for "robot nurse," or "robot butler," you'll find that a bunch of companies and universities are developing specialized (humanoid) robots to help people around the home.

For example, you'll find dozens of articles from 2004 about how Carnegie Mellon University was developing and testing Pearl the nursebot, a humanoid robot designed to help seniors with mobility and memory. This robot would talk to you, interact, and help you navigate through a crowded room. Then around 2006 the trail went cold. No more mention of poor Pearl.

There are a few other humanoid robots currently for sale. For example, Wakamaru is a domestic robot costing $14,000. It can connect to the Internet and communicate with limited speech. But as it still travels on a wheel base, its mobility is limited.

It seems that the technology is close to giving us the helpful humanoid robots we dream of, but cost is still prohibitive.

Let's give it another 10 years and check back.

Additional Resources

L earn more about Senior Technologies from the following resources. I know I sound like a broken record, but this book is just the tip of the iceberg. There are thousands of other organizations and publications out there dealing with this topic. If you're curious—which as a Senior Sleuth you most certainly are—there's a lot more to investigate. Google the topics in this book to learn more about what interests you. Get sleuthing!

Senior Organizations with Information on Technology

AARP	www.aarp.org
Center for Aging Services Technology (CAST)	www.agingtech.org
Technology Research for Independent Living (TRIL)	www.trilcentre.org

Senior Websites and Blogs

Here are a few websites that provide excellent information or services for the senior community.

✓ www.seniorjournal.com

✓ www.suddenlysenior.com

✓ www.assistivetech.net

✓ www.ageinplacetech.com
    Aging in Place Technology Watch, which features expert Laurie Orlov's
    excellent blog.

✓ www.gilbertguide.com

✓ www.robotadvice.com

✓ www.silverplanet.com

✓ www.wikipedia.org

Technology Books for Seniors

There is a growing body of how-to literature specifically for the senior
community. Here are some popular instructional titles for using computers
and the Internet. The reviews are generally positive on all of them.

✓ Computers For Seniors For Dummies (For Dummies (Computer/Tech))
    by Nancy C. Muir and Sir Stirling Moss

✓ Macs For Seniors For Dummies (For Dummies (Computer/Tech)) by
    Mark L. Chambers

✓ Using the Internet Safely For Seniors For Dummies (For Dummies
    (Computer/Tech)) by Nancy C. Muir and Linda Criddle (Paperback - Mar
    30, 2009)

✓ Senior's Guide To Easy Computing: Pc Basics, Internet, And E-mail
    (Senior's Guide) by Rebecca Sharp Colmer

✓ Windows XP for Seniors : For Senior Citizens Who Want to Start Using
    Computers (Computer Books for Seniors series) by Addo Stuur

✓ Internet and E-mail for Seniors with Windows XP: For Senior Citizens
    Who Want to Start Using the Internet (Computer Books for Seniors
    series) by Addo Stuur

✓ Windows Vista for Seniors: For Senior Citizens Who Want to Start
    Using Computers (Computer Books for Seniors series) by Addo Stuur
    (Paperback - Dec 1, 2006)

Epilogue: Case Closed!

Congratulations. You have cracked the case of Senior Technology. You can now go forth and spread the word—there are hundreds of gadgets and gizmos that can enrich the senior experience.

Although you've completed this book-driven investigation, there is always more sleuthing to be done—especially in the technology field.

New senior products are released each month. More information on how to use existing technologies appears on websites and blogs every day. I encourage you to embrace the Internet and continue your Senior Sleuthing.

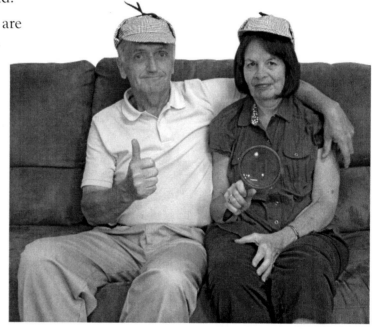

Thank you for joining me on this investigation. And now I invite you to go just a little further. Visit the Senior Sleuth website to check out our latest Senior Sleuth offerings. Make sure to leave comments and questions—especially if you use a Senior Technology not covered in this book. See you there.

Visit our website at www.sleuthguides.com.

Index

Breinigsville, PA USA
26 July 2010
242407BV00003B/1/P